D0007041

CALLED TO HEAL

humilitas

To *heal*, not to injure
To *help*, not to hurt
To *strengthen and sustain*
With *patience, compassion
and trust.*

To *unite*, not to divide
To *counsel*, not to condemn
To *reason and reconcile*
Through *peace, understanding
and love.*

God Love you

CALLED TO HEAL

Fr. Ralph A. DiOrio

DOUBLEDAY & COMPANY, INC.
GARDEN CITY, NEW YORK

Unless otherwise indicated, all scriptural citations are from *The Jerusalem Bible*, copyright © 1966 by Darton, Longman & Todd, Ltd., and Doubleday & Company, Inc.

Library of Congress Cataloging in Publication Data

DiOrio, Ralph A., 1930–
Called to heal.

1. Spiritual healing.   2. DiOrio, Ralph A.,
1930–   . I. Title.
BT732.5.D56   1982   234'.13
ISBN 0-385-18226-0
Library of Congress Catalog Card Number 82–45354

TO ALL MY FRIENDS,

Both known and unknown, who through sincere and earnest efforts, have shared with me the spirit of prayer, perseverance, and compassionate love to a world in search of the Divine Healer. As the spirit moves where He wishes and in the manner in which He wills, may He use the poverty of my words to enrich you with the meaningful wealth of His message. I bless you in His Holy Name

✝

Fr. Ralph A. DiOrio

CONTENTS

Contents

PREFACE

In the main entrance of a large and famous hospital stands a beautiful heroic-sized statue of Our Lord with the title "Christ the Healer." Not far away is a Catholic hospital with a statue of Christ the Divine Physician. On the heights of a great mountain in South America rising between Argentina and Chile stands a monumental statue of Christ of the Andes; it is a symbol of peace between the nations. Around the world, from Rome to Greece, from France to Russia, from the Orient to Africa, in churches and in homes there have been erected statues of Christ in all of His representations: Good Shepherd, Man of Sorrows, Christ the King, even one as Christ the Teacher.

But for each and every one of us I believe the most attractive and meaningful image of Our Lord is that which represents Christ as Priest. What we venerate and admire in Christ the Priest we ourselves receive from Him in the sacrifice of love on the Cross. As pastor of souls, this High Priest, Christ, nurtures us with spiritual powers of life. By the exercising of authentic and valid authority, by preaching the gospel, by teaching the truths of catechism, by especially celebrating the memorial of His agape, man becomes healed.

It is a privilege to be a priest, a minister, or a rabbi. St. Paul himself has proclaimed that to serve is to reign, and so it is that we who are called to be Christ's or God's representatives are privileged to serve. Each of us who have been called to serve our communities spiritually is called to this high dignity for no selfish purpose, but for others. "Every high priest has been taken out of mankind and is appointed to act for men in their relations with God." (Heb. 5:1) God, through His Christ, pointed out this truth when he explained the end for which the priest's work is destined, by comparing him to salt and light. The priest is the light of the world, the salt of the earth. It must be made clear to the eyes of the world that those called to serve are they who must proclaim the truth of Christianity and thus be CALLED TO HEAL.

For some time now, personages from various walks of life have sought me to expound publicly to them the "inner resources of my soul," which is the foundation of my mission as a healing evangelist. When conducting missions or evangelizing crusades, given the nature of these programs as well as time limitations, I prefer to focus on the salvation message. Rather than spend a great deal of time in describing or portraying individual gifts, my main concern is to know and speak about the knowledge of Him Who is GIFT. All else is secondary—stepping-stones to the mission of preaching and teaching about Jesus Christ as Lord.

The tappings of my soul are nothing else but the soul of the apostolate; namely, Christ and all that He stands for, Christ in His suffering and pain, Christ in His patience and perseverance . . . Christ on the cross; Christ and His blood; Christ and His seven last words. To minister Christ efficiently and adequately, one must be like Christ, live like Christ, talk like Christ, walk like Christ. One must be what the contemporary neurotic world has attempted to obliviate: *alter Christus.*

The explanation of charisms is very simple. It is that Christ must personify Himself and be experienced through those gifts of which St. Paul speaks in Romans, Corinthians, and Ephesians. (Rm. 8, 1 Co. 12, Ep. 4:11) He who would be the extension of Christ through charisms must experience no self-identity crisis. Not if he has been called by Christ. His identity to Christ has no room for a double agent. If human weakness may discourage us through vicissitudes and trials of daily activity, if the ministerial standard becomes befogged, our consolation is not in the escapisms of a self-identity crisis but in the promise of Jesus, the High Priest, Who has called us to the duties of offering sacrifice, of blessing, governing, preaching, and baptizing. Our loyalty in spite of weaknesses becomes the raw substantial material that Christ uses to keep us both humble and highly exalted. The Lord commanded Moses to choose as his helpers seventy men from the whole tribe of Israel, to whom He would impart the gifts of the Holy Spirit. He said to him: "Gather . . . men you know to be the people's elders and scribes." (Nb. 11:16) Christ in the new law chose His apostles and disciples. As He taught them whom He called, so does He call us and teach us that by word and by deed we, the ministers of His people, should be perfect both in faith and in works, that our lives should be founded on the twofold love of God and neighbor. The responsibility that flows from this injunction is that daily, whether we are up to par or not, we must strive that by God's grace we be truly worthy of having been chosen to serve God's people, His Church.

To sustain our calling with loyalty, authenticity, and responsibility, each one of us has been gifted with the very same source that Jesus Himself exercised. That is prayer. Prayer is the only answer to ministry or to mission. Nothing else; there is no substitute. A man or woman called to serve God's people must be a personification of prayer, both publicly and privately. Though my reading audience is varied as to denomination, culture, background, creed, the foundation of prayer still remains the same rock for efficient service. Being a priest, I can only express those experiences that are appropriate to my respective calling. Yet it remains true that all persons are precious before God. God needs them. God calls them by name. God sends them in His name to serve without reservation, to love without fear, to embrace without distinction.

Being a priest, I speak as a priest. Thoughts produce actions. The thoughts of my priesthood cause me to emanate the behavior of a priest in union with Christ the High Priest. For this reason, a priest who is a man of prayer brings that same spirit to his liturgical prayer life: the Mass, Divine Office, and administration of the sacraments. He brings himself as priest in his official mission to the Church. He stands before the Church as an intermediary between his people and God. In his private devotions, meditation, spiritual reading, he is perfecting his own soul and thus provides new motives for his work among the people. Through his personal prayer, Christ, Who speaks daily, every second of the day, with His chosen one, revives convictions that have probably grown weak by the stress and pressure of contemporary living. With Christ before him through a life of prayer, the exalted dignity of the priesthood of Jesus Christ will continue to spark and to energize this chosen vessel, in both his public and his official prayer life.

In the chapters that constitute this book, I have exposed to you the secrets of my soul. I can speak only of what transpires between God and me. I cannot speak of another person's transactional experiences between himself and his God. My background and my personal tendencies must be fed by their proper cravings. For me, nothing else works for the successful mission I have been called and sent to. For me, prayer works. And because prayer works for me, God the Father, through His Holy Spirit, has permitted me to experience the joys of my priestly calling: TO GIVE THE LOVE OF CHRIST.

THIS, I BELIEVE, IS THE ESSENCE OF ONE'S

CALL TO HEAL

Fr. Ralph A. DiOrio
June 1, 1982

CALLED TO HEAL

1

THE APOSTOLATE
TO THE SICK

> To those who believe,
> no explanation is necessary.
> To those who do not believe,
> no explanation is possible.
>
> FRANZ WERFEL
> The Song of Bernadette

"Infirmus eram, et visitastis me."
"I was . . . sick and you visited me." (Mt. 25:36)

Our Blessed Lord, the eternal High Priest, serves as a primary model
in the care of the sick. St. Luke, a physician himself prior to his call
to the Church of Christ, describes Jesus as the perfect example of the
Divine Physician. Most of His miracles—two thirds, in fact—were
worked to heal the ailing and one third to teach and preach. The
gospels do not record all the healings that Our Lord performed.
John the apostle himself says: "There were many other signs that
Jesus worked and the disciples saw, but they are not recorded in this

book. These are recorded so that you may believe that Jesus is the Christ, the Son of God, and that believing this you may have life through His name." (Jn. 20: 30–31) And so we have in history's biblical accounts only a partial record of the great healings, signs, and wonders that Jesus performed during the approximately three and a half years of His public ministry. But the factual accounts definitely indicate that Jesus was deeply concerned with physical healing, to which He dedicated a tremendously large part of His time. Finally, His healing power was a virtue that could deal with every kind of disease. So many personages felt Jesus' healing power: servants, children, a mother-in-law, countless lame, blind, and deaf— all who needed His healing virtue. In the gospel records there is no instance of Jesus' ever refusing to heal a wounded seeker.

Having given the example of His own behavior to the sick, Jesus required compassionate love toward the afflicted from those who were there to follow Him. The love of the sick is expected both of Christians and of religiously dedicated men and women.

The service of the sick is considered as a vocation. It is a sublime vocation, a corporal and spiritual and psychological work of mercy. It is a sublime calling because by it the commandment of charity is perfectly fulfilled. Moreover, Our Divine Saviour Himself is served in the person of the sick. When we serve the sick, we penetrate the peripheral portals of the flesh and we find the *love that waits for us*— *Christ*.

One of the most intense tragedies of human existence is the anguish of pain; far surpassing that is wasted pain. Pain with its multiple definitions, with its host of applications is still, nevertheless, no respecter of persons. It honors no distinctive status, no personage renowned or unrenowned. Pain, like a thief, like the sharpness of a surgeon's scalpel, strikes acutely, surprisingly, positively. The great and the small, the rich and the poor, the weak and the mighty, the gentle and the harsh—there are no strangers to this unwanted intruder. Pain can be wasted, and therefore fatally despairing. Or pain can be utilized and therefore become constructively enriching. Be that as it may, pain and trial will inevitably visit every human being. There is personal pain, with its own individual sensitivity. There is global pain, with its worldwide implications.

Recently, I have been deeply sensitized to that distinctive holy man dressed in white over in Rome. That human vestige filled with

God's Divine Spirit, that "*alter Christus,*" that living martyr of a broken humanity, that man, Karol Wojtyla, who came from a far-off country, now reigning in the person of Pope John Paul II, has much sensitivity to share. During his whole life he was assiduously schooled in suffering. It is both interesting and inspiring to see how this man deals with pain. It is even more uplifting to see how this man transforms the pain and anguish of human exposure to a world that at times can be cruel into Christian stepping-stones for a better tomorrow and, ultimately, an eternal bliss.

Many people, like this holy man, John Paul II, often do not refer to their pain in their apparently joyful and carefree moments. But pain dwells within them, nevertheless. Bearing it in union with God and for the benefit of mankind is a characteristic that produces saints of God.

There are times when it is necessary to speak of pain and anguish in order to disclose an inner voyage of discovery concerning the problem of pain. At still other times, it is feasible to encourage others to deal with pains of all sorts. In fact, "suffering" is a word that John Paul II uses often. If anyone can teach a wounded world about suffering and trial, about pain and anguish, from firsthand experience, it is the Holy Father.

His reign as Pope in our day is a priesthood forged in the dangers and tragedies of his beloved Poland. If we read the various accounts of his life, we see how often he risked his life for the simple freedoms we take for granted. He is a man well acquainted with danger, poverty, and physical injury. The impressiveness of his character is that he was able through Christian virtue to transform the ugliness of suffering into the sparkle of joy. With his heart and mind at one, with his focus on the Christ of his vocation, he became empowered to transform his life's trials into an alchemy of salvific benefit. God had granted the tools to do so: namely, joyful, meditative, quiet moments of prayer, Word, and sacrament.

Every true calling, if it is to have any value for oneself or for humanity, must be followed firmly and courageously. It must focus beyond the peripheral objective pain to its proper purpose. In all the pages of history, no pain has ever made a man better; but a man can be made unique in his pain! In order to escape pain, many people look to the multiple sources of relief. They seek its lessening or its complete abolishment. Many others zero in beyond this world of

daily consumption and decay. They are motivated by absolute principles that are not traitorous to the human condition. In so doing,
many turn to God. They experience this God through His visible
signs and wonders disclosing to them the answers and the remedies
of a broken humanity—a humanity that reflects all forms of pain.
Many in their anguish hear the voice of God speaking to them.
Many, too, would never have had time for God's voice if it had not
been for the intrusion of pain into their lives. St. Paul himself has
written that God has permitted that I, too, should feel in my own
flesh, suffering and weakness.

Are there not many of us who can identify with this? Illness is
generally considered as one of the most tragic temporal evils that
can befall man during his earthly voyage. Its effects are multiple,
affecting the areas of one's soul, spirit, and body. For this reason,
compassion turned into positive care is a great act of loving-
kindness. It is a work of mercy. When visiting the sick, one consoles
them as far as possible, seeking to alleviate their anguish and pain.
So very often our heartfelt sympathy shown to a sick person becomes so comforting and soothing that, from it alone, such a sick
one derives great relief and, at times, full healing or restoration.

Whenever a human being is summoned to experience suffering,
God will not leave him an orphan. The Lord will console him and
assist him either directly or through some visible agent, usually His
chosen friends. In so doing, one derives power to survive hardship on
earth and to transform it into grace, a stepping-stone to the eternal
encounter with God. One can, for example, be taught to cry prayerfully: "I invite You, my Jesus, to offer my trials with Your trials, my
anguish with Your anguish, my blood, my sweat, my tears with Your
tears, Your blood, Your sweat. And through Your Cross, Lord Jesus,
I can realize great things."

One of the most enriching experiences, is sharing oneself with another human being. It can be a voyage of discovery. A stranger becomes a friend. God's greatest gift, next to life itself, namely, supportive friendship, is revealed. In such a union two persons
communicate to each other the intensity of their inner selves. When
one is in pain, the soothing hand of a nurse, a doctor, a priest, a
friend becomes the hand of compassion. Precious indeed is this interpersonal relationship: Precious and invaluable, irreplaceable is
this call to heal the brokenhearted, the spiritually destitute, the

physically decayed. Indeed, blessed is the corporal work of mercy through the apostolate to the sick.

The apostolate to the sick is nothing else but attending the sick with whatever capacity we can, in whatever our vocation. We bring our total selves to this precious moment. Beautiful, never forgotten experiences ensue as this new interpersonal relationship unfolds. God needs external agents to speak to, to touch, other human beings. We can console the sick, teach them the Christian purpose to pain in such a manner as to offer their own sufferings for their own sins and the sins of the world, offer insight into the will of God and intercession for another's conversion and new birth experience. The offertory of one's life, consecrated with the Christ, can produce a communion of souls on earth still capable of aiding the poor souls in Purgatory. Truly, there are so many ways God can use each one of us to bind up all sorts of human wounds caused by sin, accident and disease, and by frustrated interpersonal relationships. Moreover, one can perceive that God will use him at times as a stepping-stone in preparing a terminally sick person for a happy departure from earth's life—death to this world, life in the next—the great healing.

It has always been a conviction of mine that we as priests should frequently meditate primarily on our sublime calling. The words of our ordination ceremony become, year by year, more enforcing ("Know what you do: Imitate what you minister"). They become a haunting principle of emphatic annunciation. They animate those who are sensitive to Christ's voice to live up to their ideals. This principle will console us with reassurance of our salvation. It will bring forth for all involved a rich harvest of souls to the throne of the Divine Physician.

In the service of the apostolate to the sick, the greatest beneficiaries of our attentions and ministrations are the sick themselves. When we see a fellow creature suffering, ordinary sympathy prompts us to do for him what, in a similar situation, we would look for on the part of others. That is to say, we have the opportunity and the grace to hold out to him a helping hand. Our Lord Himself assures us that He will consider every act of love rendered to the sick as true service to Himself. Now, if we ever hear of someone being ill, it should affect us as if we knew our Saviour Himself to be ill. When we are about to visit and minister to the sick, we should strive, as it were, to supernaturalize our motivation and behavior.

We should first represent to ourselves that it is Jesus Christ with whom we visit, whom we console, to whom we give assistance. Would we give to Jesus any less compassion than we would give to the black man, the Oriental, the Italian, the Frenchman, the Irishman, the German—any mere man? If we do it to Christ, one of His titles to everlasting bliss will echo forth: "I was sick . . . and you visited me." (Mt. 25:36) "I tell you solemnly, insofar as you did this to one of the least of these brothers of mine, you did it to me." (Mt. 25: 40)

Furthermore, in ministering to the sick themselves, another group of important persons are blessed; these are the rest of the household. Because of our attention, compassion, concern, and love—because we have rendered our time to those for whom time had become meaningless—there now reign light where darkness was, peace where anguish pained, insight where vision was blurred. It is a truism that people never forget what we do for their sick. In return, we see them being influenced quietly and learning to know and love again, without bitterness and resentment. They are strengthened in the faith. Often, too, some in the family who are fallen away are moved back into the Lord's embrace. Again, from the example of Jesus touching and healing, before teaching, we see countless people following the compassionate Healer and accepting His teaching *simply because* of His kindness to the sick. Jesus' example should be, even in our day, the opening wedge to win over suffering humanity to the sweet yoke of Christ.

Finally, we ourselves who minister also receive many rewards: joy and peace, as well as humility that God has used us to extend His person to another human person in search of identity and purpose. Virtues resting quietly within one who is dormant, covered with dust, inactivated by inertia, suddenly bloom again: These are compassion, sympathy, tenderness. What really is emerging is the power of the Trinity utilizing us to perform corporal works of mercy.

God's body is His Church. Christ is the Head of that Church. We are His members. The Church acts in the name of Christ. The Church has always honored these works of mercy as the highest of labors. The Church herself has shown throughout the centuries the way to practice these virtues. She herself has grown through great pains and sacrifice, charting many courses at immense expense to build hospitals, nursing homes, leprosaria, orphanages, clinics, and countless other agencies.

The Church's interest has always been to identify closest with the mind of her founder, Christ. Her thinking has been directed by the Holy Spirit to identify with Christ Himself as seen in the unfortunate, the sick, the homeless. All service so done is considered by Our Lord Jesus as truly done to His person.

If we were to verbalize the apostolate of prayer to the sick, I believe it would be: "Heal us, O Lord, and bring us together." As we mortals gaze out upon this world of creation, we see many beauties; nevertheless we must also fall upon our knees and with aching hearts shed tears for its disfigurements. Christ, Who took upon Himself the pain of man, hangs on the cross as an outcast of heaven and earth.

Endless minutes drag into eternal hours. With all the agonies of a Roman scourging and with all the horrendous inflictions of a crucifixion, Christ cries a manly cry. In His wounds, in His sores, He fears to be forgotten by men. A scream screeches like a bolt of lightning: He voices His fifth message from the pulpit of the cross to a broken and indifferent humanity: "*Sitio*—I am thirsty!" (Jn. 19:28) This pitiful screech pierces the stillness. Through bloodshot eyes, even crusted with dried blood, He gazes out on that jeering mob. His arms have been outstretched for many hours of this strange day of deicide, this Good Friday. He sees rejection by those who needed to be healed. He experiences desertion by those who should follow Him. He was delivered into the hands of strangers as an outcast in public disgrace by those who should embrace Him. He was left hanging between heaven and earth, when earth itself should have housed Him as heaven's guest. He was laughed at by those He loved. His cry, piercing as it echoed, was nevertheless a cry of a Wounded Healer in search of wounded seekers. His thirst was a cry for communion, an agonizing cry for unity. It was a cry for touch, for a caress, for a consoling word, for oil on one's bleeding wounds. It was a cry for new life, a new chance, a rebirth. He suffered on that cross. What sort of love is this: this love that submits to tortures so fearful? Where shall we find a name for it? It must be the apostolate of prayer for healing.

Writers of the past and writers of the present proclaim that thirst is by far more painful and tormenting than hunger. This is especially true with reference to anyone suffering from diminished or weakened physical strength. Jesus Himself had suffered all this anguish to an uncommon degree. He had sweated blood in the garden. He had lost a great quantity of blood upon the cross, and to add to this, His sacred body was exposed to the sun and the air as He hung there nakedly crucified. He was a stranger to sleep that day; He was tormented internally with pains and so, therefore, without any doubt He experienced a most burning thirst. Fever arising from His wounds was the principal cause of His thirst. Jesus, on the cross, experienced, then, both a bodily thirst and a spiritual thirst. He thirsted for the physical brokenness of man, as well as for their spiritual return to His Father through Him, as a prodigal son.

2

TO BE CALLED
IS TO BE CHOSEN

*At the moment that He took leave
of his apostles He commanded them,
and through them the whole Church,
each one of us: to go out and bring
the message of redemption to all
nations.*

POPE JOHN PAUL II
homily at Grant Park
Chicago, Illinois
October 5, 1979

"Here I am! I am coming to obey your will." (Heb. 10:9)

In my previous book, *The Man Beneath the Gift,** I indicated that
each soul has its own story to unfold. Each person's life, as complex
as it may be, is nevertheless rich. God has granted man human life
not by chance but for being and for purpose. As I mentioned in the

* New York: William Morrow & Company, 1980.

Introduction of that book, God has granted man his existence to mature in harmony with the Creator of all birth, of all life. If this be so, then the unfolding happenings of each man's life are nothing less than the blooming of a human soul according to the purpose of God's Divine Providence. When the Divine Creator summons a man to a vocation, He predisposes the circumstances and events of that person's life.

Does God call you and me? The answer is in the history of God and man: Saints and sinners alike have been called through many ways and many events. For example, St. Bernardine of Siena in his *Sermon on St. Joseph* (Sermon 2) speaks of God's gifts to men: "It is a general rule of God's dealing with man that when he chooses someone for special grace or some sublime role, He gives in abundance all the gifts which the person and his office require." Another example is that of St. Bernard. "Bernard, wherefore didst thou come hither, and wherefore didst thou leave the world?" These were the words, this was the question frequently placed to him when his vocation to a special calling would be tested by every kind of human storm. Such was the question St. Bernard accustomed himself to pray over when he felt the need for encouragement and strength to follow his sublime call. With God's grace, with his own determined will, with love as the furnace of his zeal, Bernard was intent never to falter from the rugged path to sanctity. He had been called to personal holiness and to ministerial service. His response was a generous surrender of earthly possibilities, possessions and honors.

A call is nothing else but a response to the sharing of one's faith in the service of others. When it is done for merely the love of man alone it is philanthropy. When it is motivated by the love of God it becomes a divine calling, an extension of God's love to man. In truth, it is the unveiling of a divine romance. St. John reminds us of this when he says: "You did not choose me, no, I chose you; and I commissioned you to go out and to bear fruit, fruit that will last." (Jn. 15:16)

Since the time that my autobiography was published, I have received many requests to share through another book the inner secrets and thoughts, the spirit and soul, within the power of the gifts of the healing apostolate of prayer and intercession for the sick.

On June 1, 1982, I had the privilege of celebrating my silver jubilee as a Roman Catholic priest. God has allowed me to serve His people as a healing evangelist. I can truly say, in spite of many hardships on the road of this mature calling, I have remained zealous. Never did I say no to the God Who called me. And because of this yes to God, all that sprung forth from my being flowed unreservedly from my whole heart and soul. With God's grace, I acquired professional-guidance degrees in the humanities and philosophies of psychology and social work, and certifications in languages and areas of spiritual theology. Other opportunities came my way as pastoral needs warranted: such as pastoral offices of all sorts, engagements in mission and retreat works, youth ministries, radio and other communication enterprises.

About six years ago, precisely May 9, 1976, God, the Author of all life and gifts, blessed me with a very beautiful charism, the gift of His healing love. It was through the Lord alone, the Lord's love for His people, that He called me in the humility of my nothingness to further priestly responsibility. He was introducing me to a tremendous ministry of mediator between Himself and a broken humanity in need of holistic renewal. He had asked me to surrender myself to make a full, self-sacrificial commitment to a life of total love and sincere compassion for a wounded humanity. I was to use His tools of prayer, teaching, Word, and sacrament.

While this ministry is by far the most demanding that I have ever had, the most exhausting of anything that I have ever been requested to do in my lifetime, it is, nonetheless, so natural because it is an authentic calling by God, provided and sustained by His grace. It is Christ extending Himself through charism to His beloved people, His broken body, His Church.

Divine strength, said Thomas Merton, is not usually given us until we are fully aware of our own weaknesses. I can still hear, echoing across the years of my formation and throughout my priestly years, that sonorous and most intent voice, so influential and inspiring that of Archbishop Fulton J. Sheen: "One becomes weary in one's work, not of it." I feel like that many times. But being called to priesthood, I presume every priest feels this way. With my brother priests who do the labor of the day I cry prayerfully: "In the midst of Your people, O Lord, I shall be love. Help me, O Lord, to teach the beauty of Your ways so that yearning souls may find You, the Christ; and they, in turn, will witness You to others."

Every vocation comes from God. Every calling is His pure gift. When God calls a person, He is choosing him. And in choosing an individual, He is loving him. When God and man meet in this calling, there is a union of complete love.

A vocation calls us to love. We invite the Giver of life to unfold the way of love, which leads us to personal fulfillment and gives our lives a purpose. In essence, a vocation is a call that God addresses to a person in the form of a special grace. The person so gifted senses it internally, because a genuine vocation inclines a person to embrace the life that the Author of life has intended for him.

During vocational psychology studies I learned that this internal feeling is called "an imperious inclination." This indicated that such a person was internally disposed by natural endowments to serve a social need, to work for the benefit of the community. In fulfilling this social service, the person discovers the essence of his or her *being*, rather than the pride and self-contentment of a camouflaged *achieving*. Happiness and joy, a sense of self-contentment and fulfillment, are personally attained. The community at large is enriched.

There lies in each individual who is called, the necessary aptitude for the work he is called to do. The dictum of the scholastics expresses this well: *"Gratia supponit naturam"*—i.e., grace works on nature. The concept of grace from God supposing and working upon nature, which is our human potential, is one of the fundamental ingredients of anyone's calling, including my own. The gift, meaning grace, really is distinct from nature. In no way does it belong to nature. Thus grace remains a totally beautiful and pure gift of God to nature. What does the gift do? It simply allows man to share in the divine nature and the divine life. This, in substance, is how I perceive the gift of healing which I received. Miraculous healing consists in a striking interposition of divine power by which the operations of the ordinary courses of nature are overruled, suspended, or modified. Incidentally, in reference to the other charisms such as prophecy, evangelism, tongues and interpretation, shepherding, or what have you, the same dictum and the concept of God's grace acting on nature applies.

St. Thomas Aquinas clearly affirms that while grace is necessary to heal wounded nature, its primary function is "to elevate nature to a share in the Divine Nature." (ST 1a, 95, 4 ad 1) Grace is supernatural. Rooted in nature, it makes nature transcend itself. St. Thomas, moreover, affirms that every conscious person possesses this capacity for elevation. Simply put, "grace elevates nature." In other words, grace builds upon and works upon one's natural potential.

If we reflect on this, we can see that every man's life from conception onward becomes the framework, the essence, the fertile soil for receptivity of God's will. All that is required, after one has been prepared by nature and tempered by life's experiences, is that at a certain moment there be total surrender to the divine plan. This point is reached, more often than not, after one has really and profoundly been humbly broken.

A person summoned by God to whatever charism, is gifted by nature itself. He is endowed with certain necessary powers in the forms of qualities and goals. Working upon these elements, God grants wounded man, through Christ, an opportunity to be healed spiritually, psychologically, and physically. This is holistic healing—healing the *whole* man.

For example, in my calling to the healing ministry, as in every other person's calling that is distinctive, what happened was that when God judged the moment right, I heard His voice, responded to His call, and stepped out in faith by surrendering to the divine plan. That which we are from nature's gift becomes nothing else but pliable clay in the Master Workman's creative hands. Thus healing, prophecy, teaching, shepherding, knowledge, wisdom, discernment, miracles, tongues, and interpretation—all the charismatic gifts, and any other natural gift a person bears within himself or herself, as sanctified by grace—reveal themselves as God's presence to a broken body in need of being made whole. Without understanding this process, trying to grasp a calling to a distinctive ministry is unintelligible and futile. God works on what He endows.

A pure call is not an occupation. A pure vocation flows from a person as naturally as the act of breathing. Feeling at ease with one's proper charism does not, however, preclude discomforting experiences. Once, for example, as a young priest in parochial work, I had to go to the house of a woman who was terminally ill. As I walked into a darkened, dismal flat with the stench from a cancerous body permeating the air, I became fearful. I myself had been physically sick for about six years during seminary training as well as for the first four years of priesthood, due to a contagious disease contracted from a former foreign student. The memory of its pain and long years of anguish had somewhat stifled my ministerial performance. So I was afraid of disease. Yet I felt very sorry and compassionate for people with sickness and disease. I was afraid to touch anything a sick person had touched. But, worse than anything else, I was afraid to touch a diseased human body. Still, I was a priest. As I was forcing myself to touch this cancerous woman, this broken human representative of a wounded Christ, the vision of Simon of Cyrene haunted me. In that one flickering of a memory, the voice of Christ hammered into my brain and heart. The Master spoke: "Ralph, it is I residing in this sick woman. Do you love Me?" Placing my heart and my emotions into the mind and heart of the Wounded Healer, I smiled gently and compassionately at the dying woman. Words so gentle and compassionate poured out of my lips: "May I pray with you, may I sit next to you, may I hold your hand? Speak to your God through me. Receive His blessings of forgiveness and compassionate anointing." So I took the holy oils; I anointed her forehead, her eyes, her nostrils, lips, ears, and feet in the sacrament of the sick. I now was touching the brokenness of humanity so diseased, as so many of my brother priests do. Christ is so near when we look for Him.

There was another incident, I recall, of a lady who had approached me with a hideous skin cancer that had eaten away part of her nose. I looked at her with deep compassion, embraced her hands in mine, and spoke to her: "Do you wish me to bless you? May I touch you? May I anoint you with blessed sacramental oil?" She answered with a pleading, beseeching: "Yes, please do." So I just held my hands there and prayed with her—her pain became mine.

On another occasion I recall a young man, approximately the age of twenty-one. Life appeared to have been harsh with him. Nature, too, was not too kind in the formation of his face. There was total disfigurement. One eye bulgingly protruded; it was the only eye he had. His mouth and nose were 75 percent turned to the left, face ballooned, rotund. At such a sight, the normal eye of an observer would naturally cringe and turn away with a repulsion and perhaps even the sensation of regurgitation.

Yet, Christ dwelled within these human beings. Christ was calling these persons to the touch and blessing of His own healing love and compassionate mercy. These incidents are very personal. The answer to their pain can only be found in the depths of a human soul. My soul speaks to God of such anguish beneath the gift. How can one sincerely speak of having been chosen to nurse a broken humanity without first having spoken of what dwells within the very core of one's soul? Furthermore, how can one adequately speak without self-revelation?

In preparing to write the present book, I was initially reluctant to express the journey of my soul with my God. Is it not true that man's greatest treasure is the secrecy of his inner being? No man should invade the delicate, gentle conscience of another human being without invitation. Nonetheless, many questions arise as a result of God's endowing me with a special calling in the Apostolate of Prayer for Healing. Rather than reduce myself to a mere computer programmed for healing, or be dubbed by a title that is so misleading, "faith healer," it would be best for the reader to perceive my life and its calling in its true reality: namely, a mere channel, a tool, a bridge by which the Father in heaven can reveal Himself to man through Jesus Christ, Who, in turn, imparts the Holy Spirit.

I can see now as I reminisce over the past fifty-two years—from the very beginning of my life, from conception, infancy, childhood, youth—how all the elements of my vocation were derived. During those early years, strong and permanent habits were formed; deep and lasting impressions were made. The direction my life would take was set. I would give it completely to Christ, with no reservations. My call to the priesthood was a natural consequence of the inner life of Catholicism and the spiritual training to which I had been exposed from my very cradle. Whatever victories and conquests God has allowed me to achieve have been done through toil and trial, through prayer and patience, through perseverance and penance. All these components were nourished by a simple, naïve, childlike trust in God.

Throughout my life I have been someone who was always compelled to do not only what man may do ordinarily but what I could do better and more. I inherited this characteristic from my decisive father; it was enforced by my mother's strong, determined character. Understandably, such a person arouses criticism and, without any effort to do so—but solely by obedience to the presence of God's will working through my docility to His call—I disturbed complacency. It is frequently said that the good is the greatest enemy of the better, and that the moderate religious people are the ones who most resent the intrusion of an apparent extremist. But since I am inclined to be optimistic and have great tolerance of criticism, I view even these obstacles as God's footsteps toward the completion of His eternal will for man and time.

When I reflect upon the criticisms that have come my way, I conclude, both philosophically and prayerfully, that the extremist, or anyone for that matter, with a distinctive vocation and a distinctive charism, has a very special function in the world to which God has directed him. That, to me, is the essence of a valid calling.

The philosophical principle of individuation is not a mere speculative classroom entertainment. Man is an individual, a sole distinctive person endowed by an abundantly filled Father. What man does with these gifts is his responsibility alone. But even more so, I continuously and emphatically teach that each distinctive soul must possess a developed character peculiarly his own. He must be unique! To be a whole person indicates harmony between the external expression of behavior and the inner conviction. If one is to be a man of God, validly and authentically summoned by God, such a one must uphold certain moral eternal truths. With God's graces working within man, he naturally becomes another Christ. With Christ in his heart and the Holy Spirit as the agent, such a person inspires his fellow men to a rendezvous with God.

Pope Pius XI, in speaking to the Catholic priesthood, said: "If, however, your work is to be blessed by God and produce abundant fruit, it must be rooted in holiness of life. Sanctity is the chief and most important endowment of the Catholic priest. Without it, other charisms will not go far. With it, even supposing other gifts to be meager, the priest can work marvels."

For those who are professed charismatics, it is interesting to grasp that these models constitute another affirmation that each soul is called by God to be a distinctive little cell in building up the broken body of the Church. Each soul was created primarily to glorify Abba through Jesus' gift of His abiding presence, the Holy Spirit. Essentially these gifts are nothing else but an expression of the new fresh baptism of God's Spirit to mankind, and actual grace urging all men and women toward a fuller experience of God and His mysteries.

For those of our contemporary age who know Christianity and also Catholicism as only institutions, I hope that you receive these inner secrets of my heart as a hopeful testimony. A look at the foundation of my apostolate reveals the very same substantial Church. It is just that old moods are present with new labels.

The same Holy Spirit, the agent of the sanctifying Trinity, utilizes a contemporary medium founded in the old. Unless blinded by prejudice, anyone can see that the true church of Christ, with all its elements and gifts, still fosters the love of Christ, the following of the Christ crucified, the power of the resurrected Christ, and the ministry of intercession of the ascended Christ. Love and forgiveness, furthermore, serve as the foundation of all genuine divine healing, for when Christ was performing His last healing love, He proclaimed from the pulpit of the cross: "Father, forgive them; they do not know what they are doing." (Lk. 23:34)

St. Ignatius once proclaimed: "Christianity is not the work of persuasiveness, but of greatness." Was St. Ignatius perhaps telling us that the most effective road to the Wounded Healer's love is to be found not in erudite dissertations but in tending to the day-to-day lives of our brothers and sisters walking across the breast of the earth —running, loving and servicing God in fellowship? Truly, therefore, to be called is to be chosen.

3

BE MY HANDS ...
BE MY HEART ...
WALK IN MY FOOTSTEPS

*Keep Jesus Christ in your hearts and you will
recognize His face
in every human being.
You will want to help Him
out in all His needs:
the needs of your brothers and sisters.*

POPE JOHN PAUL II

And Jesus said to them, "Follow me and I will make you into
fishers of men." And at once they left their nets and followed
him. (Mk. 1:17–18)

Everyone who presents himself to the Lord for His healing touch
will be healed exactly as the Lord Himself would want him to be restored. Anyone who ever approaches the Master and experiences His
presence will never be the same again. An actual grace of a new,

fresh baptism of the spirit innovates the "old man" into the "new."
What a tremendous experience to become what one always wished
to be: a restored person as God intended. And so it is with the
healing ministry. Each soul that crawls to the feet of the Lord will
arise renewed and healed either in body, soul, or in spiritual life, or a
combination of all three in what is known as "holistic healing." God
leads many persons to Himself through many avenues, and He will
even utilize the sicknesses of men themselves imposed upon men
through the original fall as a stepping-stone to His welcoming, rein-
stating embrace.

The main purpose of healing is to restore, to make new again.
God Himself has decreed that in the fullness of time He will restore
all things in Christ. All peoples, whoever they are, whatever they
have made of themselves, have a special place in the loving Heart of
the Wounded Healer. Christ's healing balm will reinvigorate everyone. It will, especially, provide the Holy Spirit of boldness to conquer despair. It will allow men and women to come together from
all walks of life, from various cultures, and to walk together. Encouraged and strengthened, a renewed person will take positive steps
for increasing his or her own dignity and will unite his or her efforts
toward the goals of human and moral advancement. The Author of
life has our lives in His care. He calls us to better things.

The true spirit of healing is found in its effects. The effects are for
the community primarily; and in so doing, the effects flow forth
from the gospel message. The proclamation of the gospel is the
strengthening of brothers, the consoling of the afflicted, the bearing
of witness to God's love, the pointing out to mankind of its tran-
scendent destiny.

When a person turns to the Lord for healing, the Holy Spirit, according to St. Paul, will be a "quickening Spirit." When one turns
to the Lord with honesty, simplicity and truthfulness, he or she can
be sure something is going to happen. When we are caught in the
tumult of conflicting emotions, some of which have their origin in
earlier training, God deals with us as we stumble along, ever ready to
bring us to new heights of glory and understanding.

The beauty of being healed by the Lord is that, being renewed
from within, we go forth humbly to witness to the community. We
undertake this task with reasonableness and with emotional balance,
avoiding any form of neurotic fanaticism in which we increase our

methods and forget our purpose. What we witness is the warmth of
the Master's command to love one another as He, the Christ Himself, loved each one of us. This may be very difficult at times. But
Christ Himself will help us. When we allow Him to do so, we begin
to speak to each other and to communicate with each other as
brothers of Our Lord.

During the past few years, I personally, through the ministry of
the Apostolate of Prayer for Healing, have witnessed so many impressive substantial healings take place in all forms. But the most
impressive were those of the very true *miracle of Healing* itself—that
is, spiritual renewal among men. I have seen hatred turn back upon
itself and melt away into love, the very opposite of hate. I have seen
where sadness reigned, joy became king. Where there was despair,
hope was born. Yes, in the past few years some really wonderful
things have taken place among God's people, His Church. Some of
these wonders have been happening where wonders should begin: in
the churches and in the communities. Those versed in theology recognize this wonder of wonders by the term "ecumenism." An appropriate name to describe this Christian dialogue is "interfaith fellowship." In praxis, however, what is really developing is that Christians
of every denomination are talking to each other and sharing with
each other. This is truly wonderful! By so doing we are acting as
Christians and brothers of the same Lord who was hanging on that
cross and gazing upon all of us as sinners in need of His redemptive
peace.

In the bond of brotherhood, the reality of the Cross's redeeming
love electrifies us to remove the prejudices that our divisions and isolations, our distrust and our separations have caused. We see them
in their true light, that is, something against God. Truly, this sign is
one of hope. It is the sign of the times. Its effects are wholesome for
a holistic healing of man himself and his community. Being such a
holy dynamic, it is then truly the visible sign of the Holy Spirit moving gently in our midst, moving steadily among us as THE
BREATH OF GOD. And in so doing, that beautiful Holy Spirit is
disturbing our smugness, from our self-made, egocentric world of
vanities and pride, stubbornness and jealousies, from our lonely
world. As he allows us a journey of inscape rather than escape, we
find that His Holy Spirit convicts us of ourselves. Then, resurrecting
our weak person, that very same Holy Spirit uses us to push onward

to the unity of our Lord's wishes as at the last meal on that Holy
Thursday, sitting with His twelve, He uttered prayerfully: ". . . *ut
unun sint*" (that they may be one). (Jn. 17:11 NAB)

And so when one speaks of discipleship one indicates a personal
prayer experience with God. This experience of God's presence, or
this actual special grace known as the Baptism of the Spirit,
impresses itself so dramatically, so influencingly upon the soul, that
eventually such an experience must externalize itself as a "personalis-
tic" dynamism.

Those of us called to the priestly life find this experience in the
foundation of the sacrament of Holy Orders, which imprints on our
soul the mark of an indelible character. Both priest, who shares in
the sacrament of Holy Priesthood, and laity, who share in the royal
priesthood of which St. Paul speaks, must of necessity become for
others a clear and plain sign. If persons are to be taken to Christ, as
Philip brought the Greeks to the Lord, so both Christians and
non-Christians want a sign, an indication. If a person is to be converted (influenced) to the acceptance of Christ, then our witnessing
must demand our closeness to the people only after we have been
close to the Master. Pope John Paul II in his discourse to the clergy
of Rome, November 9, 1978 (number 3: *L'Osservatore Romano*
November 10, 1978, p. 2) clearly stated: "Let us not deceive ourselves in thinking we serve the Gospel, if we dilute our priestly
charism."

In practical terms, it appears that John Paul II is implying that
the only authentic and reliable witnessing that is worth anything to
people is that done by the witnesser, or priest, who is conscious of
the full meaning of his own union with God. The influential
witnesser is only he or she who believes profoundly, who professes
his or her faith with courage, who nourishes his or her experiences
with the Lord by daily living-prayer. Moreover, the true witnesser is
he or she who from his or her own prayer life allows the apostolate
of the external to flow.

One who attunes oneself with the messages of Jesus as He spoke
on the Mount of Olives and on Calvary is he or she who will understand not only the personal message of the gospel but also its social
implications as well. He will be the one who will give signs and wonders to all those in need: the sick and the deaf, the blind and the
lame, the brokenhearted and the spiritually destitute. To speak of

discipleship, therefore, is to speak of the propagation of the faith to those not having heard the gospel, and of the propaganda of the faith. Whatever means is used, whatever sign is rendered, in the final analysis it is nothing else but to preach and teach the gospel of the Lord. Even the healing of man becomes a stepping-stone to teach and enrich the gospel of the Master.

In assisting man to know God, God Himself will utilize man's weak and sickened condition. Though God is not the author of pain, nevertheless He wills to do something about it. He will heal from the infinite merits of His atonement on the cross, applying those merits to all who hear of Him and accept Him. For this reason, God needs us poor creatures to perpetuate Himself to man both by Word and Sacrament. This I believe is the ultimate reason of healing, even though the immediate will of God is to heal man of his illnesses.

Often, those of us who have been blessed to serve the message and purpose of God through the healing charism are inaccurately called faith healers. I personally do not appreciate this title. To me it indicates a quantitative healing pertaining to dispositions of healer and healed. It seems to indicate faith on our part. If one is not healed in the expectation desired, nothing more cruel can be said than that he or she did not have enough faith. The only faith required is faith as a condition in the knowledge that Jesus is Lord and Healer, and that Jesus through the agency of the Holy Spirit will heal as He knows best. Our prayers do not change the mind of God. Our prayers keep us in tune with the Lord's will. The healer, to me, appears as one chosen to actualize the mind of God at this moment for His sick people. And in such manifestation those who merely observe or those who are recipients of healing are moved within their souls to a life of renewal.

Therefore, I repeat, one should never say to another who comes for the healing prayer that so much faith must be had or a healing will not be delivered. Faith is not to be measured in a measuring cup. God is not a bargainer. All healings, in whatever form they take, are totally in His hands alone. As for myself, as well as those endowed with similar charisms, we are solely channels of grace through whom God works His will.

Those thousands of persons who come from all parts of the country and beyond its boundaries by sea and air will have made the trip in vain if they fail to understand this one fundamental cause of healing: All healing is of God. He is the Healer. Man can heal no one. Man can help only the process of nature as, for example, the physician who prolongs life. Man can help another release his faith, as a priest or a minister may be so utilized. But it is God alone Who gives the grace of faith as well as the grace of healing.

Divine healing is accomplished by faith in God, who is Author, Sustainer, and Healer. Without faith, for example, medicine, as therapeutic as it is, would be ineffective. Without faith, moreover, one who prays for another's healing is helpless. Our Blessed Lord and Master said: ". . . you have believed, so let this be done for you." (Mt. 8:13) When two blind men approached Him and cried out, did Jesus not say, "Do you believe that I can do this?" They said: "Sir, we do." Then He touched their eyes, saying: "Your faith deserves it, so let this be done for you." So therefore one can see that faith is not the cause of healing; it is only a condition for the healing process. The cause of healing is the Holy Spirit.

When Jesus was on earth, He spent all His time doing good for people. The Acts of the Apostles (Ac. 10:38) says: "God had anointed Him with the Holy Spirit and with power, and because God was with Him, Jesus went about doing good and curing all who had fallen into the power of the devil." Jesus loved people and He was always interested in helping them. Nothing was too small or insignificant for Him to be concerned about. He would always be where the people were, where their needs were demanding. He always presented Himself as the insight to their needs and beyond their needs as a stepping-stone to the Father. Jesus didn't have much time to spend in the great human institutions of learning and technique. The Father, the Holy Spirit, and He were one. Within themselves they possessed the tremendous hall of fame. They were knowledge and they were love. So very often Jesus was on the seashore, along the docks, on the grassy plains of Palestine, in the marketplace, in homes. Jesus was, indeed, exactly where the people were hurting. He ministered to them as if their hearts were breaking. He has not changed. St. Paul in his chapter of Hebrews 13:8 reinforces this fact when he says: "Jesus Christ is the same today as he was yesterday and as he will be for ever."

And so Jesus Christ is concerned about each and every one of us in the very moment of the now. He sees and cares for each one of us with a watchful concern, and in so attending to our needs, in so nursing our wounds, the healing power of the Lord is to help man be like Christ in wholeness and in holiness. Our goal is *to know Him and to make Him known, to love Him and to make Him loved; to serve Him and to make Him served.* The disciple or pupil is he or she who learns from the Master, is impressed by the Master, is influenced by the things of the Master. In such a relationship of learning, the disciple generates respect and love for the Master. And in being so enveloped, the pupil is truly blessed by the Divine Teacher.

The disciple, then, in learning from the Master, becomes one with the Master. Christ specifically chose the twelve apostles as His first pupils for ministering to the Church. And in retaining unity with the Master, the apostles themselves appointed other disciples. In the Christian sense, the apostle is a friend of Christ who spends time in His presence identifying with Him and then goes forth to witness what he has experienced with the Master. The ambassador, on the other hand, is an accredited diplomat of the highest rank who is appointed by the one whom he represents. The messenger transmits a variety of messages. He not only remains faithful to his message but also faithfully represents the sender. The true evangelist, therefore, becomes the one selected by God to bear His Good News to men. He preaches the gospel to people primarily to Christianize them by the Good News. In the broader sense, moreover, the evangelist is really every Christian who witnesses Christianity to another. This is why Christ's command to teach all nations was meant for all His followers: "Go out to the whole world; proclaim the Good News to all creation." (Mk. 16:15)

Many who are called to serve the community of God with distinctive charisms are summoned specifically to a form of both general and particular healing. Sharing in the labors of a good shepherd, they, too, must through their respective charisms nourish the flock of Christ. This flock is in waiting both within and outside of the Good Shepherd's pasture. Having been trained in the school of Christ, I realize that we who are summoned to the Holy Orders become disciples and messengers. We are to preach and bear His exact doctrine; namely, the conviction of His truth experienced personally within ourselves. Gradually, then, we advance to become ambassadors. As ambassadors, we represent the Christ as His nuncios even though in so doing Christ continues to use our human words, our human deeds, our respective ways of life. Through us, through our humanity, the chief Shepherd fulfills His mission to extend Himself by imparting His gifts of love, mercy, healing, and salvation to His people.

What is the message that a disciple communicates? It is the same message that the first apostles and disciples conveyed to the whole world: "Yes, God loved the world so much that he gave his only Son, so that everyone who believes in him may not be lost but may have eternal life." (Jn. 3:16) What a beautiful message entrusted to all of us! I personally have never needed to change this message in order to present myself as an influential spokesman to the people. Often I am asked what is the exact message of my healing ministry, what is the ingredient I use to draw the crowds of thousands who come? I respond that it is the commission of Jesus Christ. For me, His message is not changed. It is the same for all ages. "For God sent his Son into the world not to condemn the world, but so that through him the world might be saved." (Jn. 3:17) The gospel of Jesus Christ never need be changed, only applied. The gospel is and always will be relevant in substance to every age, to every culture, to every society under any conditions.

I believe my ministry is serving the Church as a link between the old and the contemporary expressions of the Holy Spirit. From my own observation, coupled with the reflections of other sensitive observers, God appears to be using this ministry of the Apostolate of Prayer for Healing as a liaison. In essence there can never be a division between the institutional Church (better called the ancient Church) and the contemporary Church.

As I stated previously, the Church of Christ is not an organization like some political party, or a business firm, or something of that sort. The Church of Christ is an organism. It has a head, Jesus Christ; it has arteries, the apostles; it has cells, baptized Christians. Archbishop Fulton J. Sheen wrote the following in a booklet entitled *The Fullness of Christ*:

> If there is any picture which adequately describes the Church in time it is that of a person living throughout the cataclysms and revolution, the progress and the unfolding of the centuries . . . when, therefore, we in this twentieth century wish to know about Christ, about His early Church, about history, we go not only to the dusty

records but to the living Church, which says to us: "I lived with Christ. I saw His Mother. I saw Christ at Caesarea Philippi when He made Simon the Rock." It is the same Church with the same soul that gave birth to the *Paul* who was Saul of Tarsus. It is the same Spirit who led Barnabas into Germany, Augustine into England, Cyril and Methodius to the Poles, and Patrick to Ireland.

The most precious title of Jesus, to Christians, is "Saviour." That title, with all its implications, is what the Apostolate of Prayer for Healing represents. Jesus came into a world in which salvation lingered in the hearts of men as a universal and deep desire. The world, when Christ appeared in the pages of its history, was looking for salvation. Isaiah 43:1 tells us: "Do not be afraid, for I have redeemed you; I have called you by your name, you are mine." The salvation message of Our Lord Jesus Christ needed visible signs. It needed the flesh and the blood of men who would rally around the Master, Christ Himself, as only followers could gather around a leader. And so, to extend His person, the Son of God, Who had become Man, gathered unto Himself a handful of chosen men with their own respective personalities, idiosyncrasies, temperaments, and individual characteristics. With all their foibles and follies, with all their blunderings, they were, nevertheless, the first company of Jesus. The distinctive feature of this rendezvous between God and man was that Jesus, Himself, mustered unto Himself *special men.*

Who were these men whom Jesus called? They were recruits whom in His Divine Providence He would meet intentionally as He apparently wandered the sands of Palestine. Their talents were varied, their characters different, and their personalities divergent. Occupation-wise, they came from multiple backgrounds: fishermen, a tax collector, carpenters, and tentmakers. As Jesus pierced into their eyes, He read within each man the potential of tremendous possibility for service. He did not waste time at what they had made of themselves up to that moment, but He foresaw what He would make of them through His divine and human touch. And so He summoned unto Himself twelve stouthearted men equally distinctive from among many, just as He would summon unto Himself men from all ages. So at this moment, as He began to construct the bark of Peter, His Church that would weather every storm of the ages to come, He called these individual men as His exclusive delegates for the commencement of the new evangelization.

The gospel narratives themselves are so compelling that as one reads them one would be immediately willing to put all things aside to follow in the footsteps of Him whose road would lead to a new Pentecost through the portals of a resurrection preceded by a Golgotha. Any true evangelization program that follows in the blueprint of the Master will realize that the Pentecost of old and the ongoing Pentecost cost God something; it cost Him the price of His Son.

According to the narration incidents, Jesus proceeded from a deep encounter of prayer and fasting. As His footprints came forth from the desert, His sandaled feet made traces along the pathways and shores of Galilee: "On the following day as John stood there again with two of his disciples, Jesus passed, and John stared hard at Him and said, 'Look, there is the Lamb of God.' Hearing this, the two disciples followed Jesus. Jesus turned round, saw them following and said, 'What do you want?' They answered, 'Rabbi,'—which means Teacher—'where do you live?' 'Come and see,' he replied: so they went and saw where he lived, and stayed with him the rest of that day. It was about the tenth hour." (Jn. 1:35–39)

The Gospel of Mark has something even more explicit. It is beautiful in its narration. He speaks about the appointment of the twelve: "He now went up into the hills and summoned those he wanted. So they came to him and he appointed twelve; they were to be his companions and to be sent out to preach, with power to cast out devils. And so he appointed the Twelve: Simon to whom he gave the name Peter; James the son of Zebedee and John the brother of James, to whom he gave the name Boanerges or 'Sons of Thunder'; then Andrew, Philip, Bartholomew, Matthew, Thomas, James the son of Alphaeus, Thaddaeus, Simon the Zealot and Judas Iscariot, the man who was to betray Him." (Mk. 3:13–19)

What a microcosm of human potential! All that needed to be was the Master's touch, the Potter dealing with the clay. Truly, God can call everyone. All that ruminates quietly in the heart of Jesus is that those whom He calls will respond and will remain faithful and loyal to Him. The Master Himself proclaims in the words of John 12:32, "I shall draw all men to myself."

What did all these different novices have in common? That which they bore in common was a volcanic heart of true discipleship based not upon what they knew, know, or would know, but on how much they would loyally love the Master. One of the most striking features about the first group of adventurers in quest was their diversity of character. They exhibited fiery temperament, dauntless spirit and seemingly irreconcilable traits. The prophet Isaiah of old might have reflected on the possibility that these recruits of the Master would personify the vision of the wolf and the lamb. How beautifully, how uniquely, what a masterful stroke of genius and artistry the Carpenter of Nazareth performs when He polarizes opposites into togetherness for the serious business of serving God!

Again we ask, What did all these clumsy novices, exuberant and rustic, politically and socially inclined, gentle and sweet, simply humdrum, day-to-day characters, have in common? Their common denominator was that as men in search of a quest they found THE CHRIST.

The disciples of Jesus were young men, virile men, robust at times, harsh at others, melancholic, choleric, sanguine, and phlegmatic. Their temperaments and their speeds, their likes and their dislikes were truly multiple. At times they were downright boisterous, gruff. They were apostles in the raw material; each one of them in the mind of the great Potter was to be a rock of strength in the formation of the Church. Their ages ranged from approximately twenty-two to twenty-eight or thirty. A few of them, like Peter, were married. God had taken them through His Christ just where they came from. He would use their naturalistic spirit of the moment and transform it with His grace from an imprudent, irrational form of behavior to a fiery zeal with a cause. Some of these men were nationalists fighting against the Romans who had intruded in the conquest of the land of Palestine. Simon the Zealot, for example, was one of the nationalists who despised the Roman eagle. Though he was a fiery nationalist, he had been brought into the company of Jesus and is seen walking arm in arm with Matthew, the tax collector, the publican. Matthew, on his part, seeking the benefit of the moment, had sided with the Romans in order to enjoy an epicurean life-style. For the sake of the material, he had compromised his beliefs and possibly his morals.

On the other hand, we have that figure of Scripture whom all of us chuckle at. We see him as robust, intemperate, hotheaded, warm, impulsive, angry, sanguine, melancholic. We see his tremendous talent to transform a cussing remark—so apropos to a Galilean fisherman, whose nets most probably at times entangled themselves, thus angering him into impatience and impulsivity—into a sweet, gentle aspiration arrowing itself into the heart of Jesus. This man, called Peter, swearing at one moment, praying at another, melancholy at one moment, and sanguine at another, is also one who wants his country free from the burdensome yoke of an intruding Roman Empire. But again, walking in the company of Jesus, this man Peter joins with Matthew. This fiery ball of humanity, this man of energy, activity, impetuosity, is the very same man who becomes tempered by the fires of the divine love of Jesus. He, in turn, also becomes a complement to the refined, gentle, sweet John. John is meditative, thoughtful, prayerful, visionary, idealistic. His sincere life of prayer enriches him to know the human heart of a suffering Christ and the mind of his Master, Who is One with the Father. And yet that same principle which transcended them from their natural gifts into distinctive charisms was the constant: *They found the Christ*. That's what kept them together: the Christ with them—nothing else!

Then there was Andrew. Peter was his brother. Andrew comes through the pages of Scripture as a notable figure. Nothing seems to trouble his faith. The Scriptures describe his ministry as flowing from his personality. He appears to be the one who introduces everyone to Jesus. Philip, who was practical, functions beautifully with him; they both appear to serve as excellent public-relations men. As one reads the Scriptures of St. John, Chapter 1, verse 41, one is excited at the great finding of Andrew: " 'We have found the Messiah' —which means the Christ—and he took Simon to Jesus. Jesus looked hard at him and said, 'You are Simon son of John; you are to be called Cephas'—meaning rock."

Now, this Andrew with his peculiarity of being positive in his findings, staunchly adherent to faith with its disclosures, chums along nicely with the doubting Thomas. Thomas is constitutionally melancholic. Doubt is his constant companion. Touch is his constant need. His favorite words are "Prove it to me!" He is a staunch adherent of the materialistic. His pleasure is grounded in the pragmatic.

These are the first apostles whom the Lord called. As we contemplate them, could we not be among them? In this first small group we see the foundation of the universality of the Church being formulated. The unifying cement to these vessels of clay, these pebbles gathered from along the shores of the lakes, is the unifying principle of the Christ Himself. There is something about the Christ that, when we look into His eyes, His gaze will continue to haunt us until we unreservedly surrender ourselves to the Lord. Like a pebble of sand that irritates the oyster in order to produce the pearl of great price, so will the encounter of Jesus continually disturb these apostles' minds and the minds of all mankind. The memory of the Christ would always be there; His words, His thoughts, His walk, His touch, the things He enjoyed, those things which He condemned.

No tragedy would ever have the power to disintegrate their loyalty to Him even if at times the cries of their broken humanity would scream for a divine manifestation. For example, after the crucifixion tragedy, these men were terribly frightened. The fear of their humanity drew them to hide in the Cenacle like a group of frightened kittens abandoned by their nurturer. But it was Mary Magdalene, that renewed birth of love, that shattered vessel now restored, who came up and excitedly said to them, *"He is risen!"*

"What do you mean!" they exclaimed. And as they looked at each other with bewilderment, possible anger with themselves for having dispersed from and abandoned their condemned Master, possibly angry still that a woman called Magdalene should outshine them in faith, hope, and love, they argued among themselves. Anger being ventilated, they now were ready to deliberate—with their different personalities still interacting. To bring them peace and unity, Christ broke through the wooden doors of the Cenacle and there, in their midst, He appeared to them as the Wounded Master, glorified. There He was in resurrection power.

At other times during the forty days after His resurrection, some of the apostles, not knowing what to do with themselves, were returning to their old ways of life. And so it was that the Christ again appeared to them eight times during those forty days to enrich them, to confirm them.

They had been reverting to the world to solve their problems. But it was the Christ who led them to the mountain of Olivet, where they were no longer novices of discipleship. There, upon that mountain, they became apostles and ambassadors of Him Who had called them and of Him Who was to send them: "All authority in heaven and on earth has been given to me. Go, therefore, make disciples of all the nations; baptize them in the name of the Father and of the Son and of the Holy Spirit, and teach them to observe all the commands I gave you. And know that I am with you always; yes, to the end of time." (Mt. 28:18–20)

Do you hear His call? Is the Master also calling you? As Christ called that first company of men and women to service, taking them from exactly where they were and with what they had, drawing forth from their weak humanity a restored humanity enriched with His divine grace, so, too, Jesus is summoning men and women from all ranks of life, from all ages, to the ministry of witnessing, as Christ magnetized the first apostles to Himself when He said, "Come and see"; when He said, "Follow Me"; when He said, "Come, stay with Me awhile." So He says unto you and me: "Do you wish to know Me? Do you wish to know who you are, where you are going, Who your God is, . . . then come, follow Me. Live with Me, dine with Me, speak with Me; I'll talk to you, I'll change you and, like My first novices, you in turn will go forth to change the world, and not be changed by it. Be My disciples, be My apostles; allow Me, through the instrumentality of your humanity, to become gift to mankind. Give Me your hands that I may bless and touch both you and the world. Give Me your heart that I may not only give you a new thrill to the beat of life, but that through you I may love the forlorn. Give Me your voice, that I may speak the words of divine compassion and Good News. Give Me your feet, that I may trod footsteps and pathways for the lonely wanderer and the searching seeker. Through you, allow Me, Who am the Wounded Healer, to mend the wounded seeker. I am with you all days."

Those who follow the call of Jesus find themselves His friends: "I have not called you servants, you are my friends." How thrilling to have Jesus call us friend! Jesus started out alone. He walked and taught and searched for followers. He found men who had a need to be filled. He made them His pupils. He made them His friends. Jesus thereupon molded these ordinary but distinctive characters and personalities into giant apostles. God the Creator had already endowed them with natural gifts. And in so doing, God disposed them for their primary vocation. All that was needed was their response. This would be given to them by the Christ and the Holy Spirit at the precise, opportune, divinely planned moment. Like the ring of a giant bell, the voice of Christ echoes continuously in the hearts and minds of all to whom He offers the divine invitation.

At times of discouragement and hardship—rather than being stymied, stifled and victims of inertia—it is good to recall the gospel stories of those who followed the Master, who committed themselves to Jesus.

The first apostles followed Christ with an eager "yes." They went with Jesus, following Him upon His way: Galilee, Samaria, Judea, Bethany, Gethsemane, Mount Tabor, Tiberius, *Jerusalem!* They left their boats, their tents, their businesses, promptly and without hesitation—whatever the cost to them. As they stayed close to the Master, as they walked with Him, as they remained constant in His presence, they could not help but learn more about what He expected of authentic apostles.

Anyone who walks in Jesus' company must be transformed by His presence. Once having walked in the presence of Divinity, a follower of Christ will always remain awestruck; eventually he must experience the illumination and the rays of the Mount of Transfiguration.

As for the souls of these apostles, nothing in the world could or would ever satisfy them again. The following of Christ became a passion like that of a volcano, boiling and purifying them through an inner renewal. They surrendered to the influence of Jesus, who never coerces. Rather, He influences, invites the searcher to surrender his or her age-old ache and wounded heart to Him, the Healer of all hearts. Job testifies well of this when he says: "If only I knew how to reach him." (Jb. 23:3)

Augustine himself, after twenty years of philosophical and theological quests, after countless pragmatic investigations of possible solutions to life and its mysteries, after innumerable experiences in the way of irrational behavior and immorality, surrenders to his God. With one deep sigh, Augustine cries out, with a cry that still echoes in our own time: "O God, I shall not rest until I rest in Thee." The chase and the capture are complete.

All of us, like the apostles, are called by name to follow our Leader, Jesus. Yes, even as the apostles, we, too, follow the Master into the unknown, even into uncharted waters, at times perceiving dimly Who He really is or where He is leading us. It is a journey of stepping out in faith. Haven't all of us at some time in our lives done the same?

When I heard the call of the Lord, at the early age of fourteen, I, too, did not think where I was going, nor did I dillydally about my surrender to the Lord Jesus. All I wanted was to continue to be in His presence, to do whatever He wanted me to do. I did not fuss or overburden my mind about where He was leading me. His presence was real and abiding, continuous and constant, experienced each day through prayer. I felt great joy.

The journey would apparently be long, the course would be arduous, but the grace would be given, the goal would be His. All that He required of me was that I accomplish the daily sacrament of the moment, that is, sanctify the human element of my day with His divine guidance.

As long as Christ would remain the source of my strength, my vision would be acute. I never said no to Christ, nor would I want to say no to Him in the moment of my greatest calling.

The first apostles were gripped and held by something irresistible residing in the person of Jesus. Some of their friends laughed at them. Others plotted schemes against them, and in moments of sadness, in moments of lack of self-contentment, they became angered and depressed. During such times of discouragement and despondency, they wished they were out of the whole perplexing business of following Jesus. But still they clung to Jesus. And the more they clung to Jesus the more they became like barnacles adhering to the matrix ship, the personification of loyalty, devotion, and victory.

A walk with Christ, be it short or long, is a step on the path to maturity. I am still maturing. Each one of us is still in the process of maturing, be he or she young or old, novice or expert. None of us is complete; I am not complete. Far from it. But what is wonderful is that the Christ continues to work on us as the Potter with the clay. We know our nothingness the more we experience the presence of the Lord. Like the apostles, each one of us has received a new birth through Christian renewal. All of us have been beckoned to stand beneath the Cenacle balcony to witness the manifestations of the new Pentecost. With God's hand upon our shoulders, with Christ's footprints tracing steps forward, both you and I will reach that measure of victory to which Christ and His Church summon us on.

Then as we reminisce over pages and chapters of our own autobiographies, it is consoling to see that we will have undergone the six steps to the growth of Christ once outlined by the erudite William

Barclay, of Scotland. In his booklet *The Life of Jesus for Every Man*, Barclay reflects on these steps: (1) preparation; (2) conflict; (3) recognition; (4) tragedy; (5) triumph; (6) His body, the Church, as it reigns.

I am sure that you, too, have experienced these various phases of spiritual growth, and the greatest day of grace for you—as it was for me—was the day you stepped out in faith to God, resurrecting all the graces you had received through previous sacramental blessings of the Holy Spirit. To prepare us adequately, Christ utilized His own tools of surgery. In so doing he cleared away our peripheral selves. He emptied us, both you and me, leaving us not emptied as a vacuum, but filled up with Himself, breathing into us the breath of His Holy Spirit.

As I conclude this chapter, I am reminded of a story so dramatically told by Archbishop Fulton J. Sheen in his series of cassettes *The Answers to the Seven Burdens of Life*. The entire narration seems to epitomize Christ's love alone that urges us on:

> During the crusades there was a man called Robert Bruce. Bruce wanted to go on the crusades and he felt sick and was dying. Before he died, he told his friend, Lord Douglas: "Cut my heart out and carry it with you unto the crusades." And as Lord Douglas was facing the Saracens and his men were weak, frightened, hungry and tired before the walls of Jerusalem, Lord Douglas vigorously mustered his men with a cry: "In my hands here, I hold the heart of Bruce who would will to go where he want." And he took the heart of Bruce and flung it amidst the enemy, among the Saracens, and as the heart of Bruce rested among the enemies' feet, Lord Douglas was heard to rally: "Where the heart of Bruce has gone, now we go to conquer and save the heart of Bruce." And they went in and struggled and won the battle.

And that's how it is with our fidelity and loyalty to Christ. We disciples and followers have to endure tragedy, suffering, and sorrow. But so long as Christ remains our goal, then His love, His person alone will aid us to surmount all human problems and difficulties.

So the Lord has called. How will we answer? He beckons us to His wounded side. The gaping wound of the divine heart invites us to become spiritual gate-crashers. Each drop of His blood becomes a red river that charts our vocational call. If still we feel unworthy to answer the call, then let us fall upon our knees before our crucified

Master and pray to him with the memorable words of St. Thomas à Becket:

> My Lord, Jesus, I find it difficult to talk to you. What can I say, I who have turned away from you so often with indifference. I have been a stranger to prayer, undeserving of Your friendship and Your love. I've been without honor and feel unworthy. I am a weak and shallowed creature, clever only in the second-rate and worldly arts, seeking my comfort and pleasure. I gave my love—such as it was—elsewhere, putting service to my earthly king before my duty to you. But now they have made me the shepherd of Your flock, guardian of Your Church. Please, Lord, teach me now how to serve you with all my heart: to know at last what it really is *to love, to adore,* SO THAT I MAY WORTHILY ADMINISTER YOUR KINGDOM HERE UPON EARTH AND FIND MY TRUE HONOR IN OB-SERVING YOUR DIVINE WILL. Please, Lord, make me worthy.

4

A SHEEP'S CRY,
A SHEPHERD'S SIGH

"Be the shepherds of the flock of God that is entrusted to you:
watch over it. . . ." (1 P. 5:2)

To be a shepherd means to have within oneself elements of abundance, to be shared with and ministered to those who have less abundance. In other words, to be a shepherd is to be aware of another's poverty. To be an *authorized* shepherd requires the shepherd to be willing to give up his own abundance whenever those who are less abundant call on him to do so. Thus, anyone chosen by Christ to be a shepherd, after a while becomes the personification of the "Good Shepherd," the true Shepherd, Jesus Christ.

In thinking about shepherding, I recall this story: "Once, a hungry, ragged little fellow was being taunted by a group of well-dressed older boys. 'Why doesn't God tell someone to help you?' they said. The little fellow thought for a moment, and then, with tears in his eyes, replied: 'I think He does, but nobody listens to Him.'" Isn't this sad response all too familiar?

Men who act as spiritual leaders bear a tremendous responsibility. Jesus said to Peter: "Look after my sheep." (Jn. 21:17) All men engaged in religious leadership are called on to feed their flock. The great ideal of the minister or the priest is as one who has this sense of duty toward his flock.

In my role as a priest I am also, and fundamentally, a shepherd ministering to my flock. And in this modern age of spiritual hunger and physical hurt, the flock cries out for nourishment and healing.

The idea of priesthood, of shepherding, is beautifully expressed in a little story that influenced my own life while on the road to priesthood. Although I can't recall where I first read the story, I do know it offered me firm inspiration in my strivings toward priesthood. It is the story, in figurative and poetic language, of Old Wolf, a Cheyenne Indian chief of Montana:

> In the land of the Cheyennes, there is a mountain higher than all the mountains around him. All the Cheyennes know that mountain; even our forefathers knew him. When children, we ran around wherever we wanted. We never were afraid to lose our way so long as we could see that mountain, which would show us home again. When grown up, we followed the buffalo and the elk; we cared not where we pursued the running deer, so long as the mountain was in sight; for we knew he was ever a safe guide, and never failed in his duty. When men, we fought the Sioux, the Crows, the white men. We went after the enemy, though the way went high up, and low down. Our hearts trembled not on account of the road; for as long as we could see the mountain, we felt sure of finding our home again. When far away, our hearts leaped for joy on seeing him, because he told us that our home came nearer.
>
> During the winter, the snow covered all the earth with a mantle of white; we could no longer distinguish him from other mountains except by his height, which told us he was the mountain. Sometimes dark clouds gathered above. They hid his head from our view, and out of them flew fiery darts, boring holes in his sides. The thunder shook him from head to foot, but the storm passed away, and the mountain stood forever.
>
> This mountain is the black-robe. His heart is as firm as a rock. He changes not. He speaks to us the words of truth. We are always sure of our path, when we look to him for guidance. He has taught us in the summer of his days. And even now, when his head is whitened by the snows of many winters, and his face is wrinkled by the storms of life, we still recognize him as our spiritual chief. He is the mountain that leads up to God.

Yes, the priest is the mountain, the "rock" that draws all men to rise above themselves, to look upward toward the sublime. In my mind, the priest must be another Christ; he must center his whole life around the doctrine and the spirit of Jesus Christ. It is not enough for him merely to receive, in his training, the liberal and professional education suited to his vocation. Unlike those of other professions, the priest must acquire habits of thought and character that make him the "salt of the earth" and the "light of the world."

We might say that while a doctor heals bodies, a priest heals souls; while a soldier fights for his country against other men, a priest fights for God and souls against the army of sin and hell; while a teacher trains minds for worldly success, a priest trains them for eternal happiness; while a judge may free one innocent who has been falsely accused, a priest in the sacrament of reconciliation restores innocence even to the guilty; while a policeman guards earthly treasures, a priest is keeper of the greatest treasures of all, the sacraments; while a warden can open and shut the gates of a prison, a priest has the power to open and close the gates of heaven and hell.

The priest is a fisher of men and a steward of the house of God. He is a spiritual father of many people and an ambassador of Christ. He is a shepherd of souls and a dispenser of the mysteries of God. He is a fellow worker with Christ and a sower of good seed; a hunter of souls and a bearer of good fruit. He must face the realization that his only *real identity* lies in his being another Christ, in deed and in truth.

As Christ's representative—disciple—ambassador—teacher—evangelist—healer—the priest is commissioned to do good to all men. He administers the life of Christ through the sacraments, through preaching, through the offering of the holy sacrifice of the Eucharist. He attracts all men to Christ through the holiness of his life. If the priest, the shepherd, is a saint, his people will be holy; if the priest is only holy, his people will be only good. If the priest is merely good, his people will be fair; if the priest is simply fair, his people will be mediocre. If the priest is mediocre, his people will be bad. The sheep who have no shepherd starve. As it says in Ezekiel (34:5–6,10): "For lack of a shepherd they have scattered, to become the prey of any wild animal; they have scattered far. My flock is straying this way and that, on mountains and high hills; my flock has been scattered all over the country; no one bothers about them and no one looks for them. . . . The Lord Yahweh says this: I am going to call the shepherds to account. I am going to take my flock back from them and I shall not allow them to feed my flock." (see also Jr. 23:1–5)

When I was young and thought about becoming a priest, I connected the idea of "priest" with the idea of "shepherd." Two childhood experiences helped to shape my concept of what it means to be a shepherd.

As a nine-year-old, I loved to listen to my elders. These family elders seemed to possess an innate talent for telling homespun stories and drawing from them moral lessons. My uncle, Justino, had a small farm with a goat and a sheep. When I visited him, I observed how different was the behavior of the ugly goat from that of the sheep. I much preferred the little lamb; it seemed so clean and gentle, so meek and helpless. I began to see, from my own observations and my uncle's stories, why the shepherd should take such care to look after his flock. In the fifth grade at Old Arlington School, in Cranston, Rhode Island, I had an experience that directly shaped my later concept of the "shepherd" and his role. Mrs. Corrigan, a fine Protestant teacher whom I greatly admired, would commence our school day by leading us in prayer through the recitation of the "Our Father" and Psalm 23. Each day, as we came to the termination of the "Our Father," I was keenly aware of the way the prayer ended differently for different religious denominations. I wondered why we couldn't "all be one" in speaking to God, if we really were all His children. My Protestant friends, who sat near me, added words to the "Our Father" that impressed me deeply: "For Thine is the kingdom, and the power, and the glory forever!" We Catholics said merely a simple "Amen" after asking the Lord to "deliver us from evil." We lacked these beautiful words. It made me feel inadequate and somewhat shortchanged. The impact of that moment was revealed many years later, when God, using that sharp memory of denominational difference, led me to the evangelistic trend that runs through my ministry.

At present, at my healing services, that long-ago experience colors my efforts to improve interpersonal relationships and heal persons of many denominations. Shortly after the service commences, and the entire congregation is standing, I suggest that all Roman Catholics be seated, leaving brothers and sisters of other Christian and non-

Christian families standing. Then I urge the Roman Catholics to approach and greet these brethren and in welcoming them to ask forgiveness for any possible hurts, intentional or unintentional, caused through the years. Similarly, the non-Catholics are asked to extend a reciprocal gesture of charity, seeking forgiveness of the Catholic congregants. A sense of love and peace fills the air. This coming together in forgiveness has proved to be a strongly effective means of healing. It has drawn favorable comment from clergy and laity alike. I believe that forgiveness, expressed by surrender, is indeed the foundation to healing.

When I think back on the differences between my Uncle Justino's sheep and goat, I remember noticing that they were not able to graze in the same area. Yet they survived on the same land, ate plants grown in the same earth, and drank from the same well. Puzzled, I asked myself, Why? Why could they not be one? I searched for an answer. In Scripture, does not Isaiah speak of the "lamb and the wolf"? Better still, did not Christ Himself bring unity out of the diverse characters of His chosen apostles? Truly, they were all united by that one common bond: the Christ Himself.

In Christ's identification of Himself as the Good Shepherd, "I am the good shepherd: the good shepherd is one who lays down his life for his sheep" (Jn. 10:11), He emphasizes His love for *all* men. Using the analogy of a shepherd who keeps guard over His sheep, He refers to a mutual bond of knowledge and love between Himself and all members of His body. This can also be taken as a definition of the Church, meaning the "flock" over which the Good Shepherd, Christ, presides. In His absence, Christ carries on the ministry of shepherding through His body, the Church. Just as He called Himself the Good Shepherd, so Christ calls others to be good shepherds, representing Him in attending the flock, the sheep, the Church, His people. As we read in 1 Peter, "Now I have something to tell your elders: . . . Be the shepherds of the flock of God that is entrusted to you: watch over it, not simply as a duty but gladly, because God wants it. . . ." (1 P. 5:1–2)

This is an invitation to holiness, and holiness is nothing else but surrender of the human will to the will of God. Such surrender calls for an ascetic way of life, consisting of prayer, mortification, and fasting—daily active graces that strengthen the union of instrument and cause. The true purpose of good shepherding is to become one with Christ, that Christ might walk, speak, and love through His instrument.

Furthermore, when Jesus expressed Himself as the Good Shepherd looking for sheep who were lost, He portrayed Himself as "Saviour," as Mediator standing between God and man. As He stood between God and man, He united the two natures, human and divine, in the Second Person of the Blessed Trinity.

In grasping why God became man, it must be understood that man is a limited being, while God is an infinite being. Man committed sin against the Godhead. In so doing, he insulted and infinitely offended the Creator. As a result, from a point of justice, human restitution had to be made to the Godhead. But man, in his human inadequacy, could never accomplish this in full. How could man, with his limited human power, make adequate restitution to the infinite God? How could this moral order, which had been shattered, be rectified? How could a man-and-God relationship be healed, restored, and renewed? How could man return to his God?

If a child insults a parent and then says, "I'm sorry," that would seem to be enough. The offense of insulting the parent, serious as it is, nevertheless holds not the same intensity of insult as would be the case with a person of higher status—such as the president of a country.

So man, a limited, finite being, offends an infinite, unlimited God, to Whom he could never make adequate recompense. But God, never faltering in His mercy, wisdom, and love, brings forth the Christ from a virgin whom He had prepared from all eternity: Mary. The Holy Spirit activated within her virginal womb a human nature, the Christ, the Anointed One, without the aid of a human person. This specifically is the mystery of Christmas, the mystery of the Incarnation. From the very moment of conception, the person indwelling in the child of Mary was the Word of God, the Second Person of the Blessed Trinity, now made flesh. For this reason, His humanity can laugh, smile, suffer, and totally make up for the offense of man against the Godhead. But His way of choice was the Cross. Every action that the humanity of Christ performs belongs and is attributed to the very person of Christ, that is, the Second Person of the Trinity. Therefore, the Son of God is acting in and through the human nature of Christ. In this manner, Christ justifies, rectifies, redeems, regenerates, and heals the body of the Church. He is

Saviour. He is Evangelist. He is the Ambassador of the Father, He is the Priest, and He is the Good Shepherd.

A true shepherd walks in the footsteps of Christ, as he judges, disciplines, delivers, and governs his people, feeding and making a covenant with them. Proverbs 27:23 tells us: "Know your flocks' condition well, take good care of your herds. . . ." He protects his people, blesses and establishes them. Christ Himself gives them the value of identity as they allow themselves to be assimilated into Himself.

In the areas of personal responsibility and ministry, "shepherding" takes many forms. "And to some, His gift was that they should be apostles; to some, prophets; to some, evangelists; to some, pastors and teachers; so that the saints together make a unity in the work of service, building up the Body of Christ. In this way we are all to come to unity in our faith and in our knowledge of the Son of God. . . ." (Ep. 4:11) According to Paul, we then become the perfect man, the perfect instrument, and we daily mature with the fullness of Christ Himself, so that in ministering we respect the body, the Church, and we respect the head, who is ministering properly to the body.

This is the object to which shepherding has to lead: *building Christ's body*. The shepherd's functioning pertains solely to this renewal. Furthermore, in adequately building Christ's body, the ministering individual or the ministering group bears tremendous responsibility. None of us should allow ourselves to become overexcited about the new birth we have received or about public recognition of the ministering power placed in us by God. Our sole purpose is to stay united with Christ, so as to allow the Christ to minister to His people in need. "Make your home in me, as I make mine in you. As a branch cannot bear fruit all by itself, but must remain part of the vine, neither can you unless you remain in me. I am the vine, you are the branches. Whoever remains in me, with me in him, bears fruit in plenty; for cut off from me you can do nothing." (Jn. 15:4–5) It is supernatural grace that allows each unpretentious person to recognize the natural gift that God has given him alone, and God sanctifies the natural gift when it is willingly surrendered. He elevates it to the status of charism. It is now ready for the good of man, and for the building up of the body of Christ.

In serving God's people through the ministry of healing as a priest, disciple, or evangelist, the supreme authority that functions through me is Jesus Christ. He is the authority, for He is the true "Rock" of the Church. However, for valid functioning, authority and accountability should go hand in hand. They are related to one another in essence (authority: Jesus Christ) and nature (functioning: the instrument). All of us must be accountable, for our behavior, both to Christ and to His legitimately appointed authority, who allows us the privilege of functioning in the name of the body's welfare. *My ministry functions only because it IS legitimately authorized for the welfare of the Church.* Without such acknowledgment of authority, dissension and divisiveness result. We have churches at variance with one another's dogmas, breaking off into other churches, other bodies, other ministries. That is not unity in Christ. Nor is it health for the broken body of the Church. And the flock is always the one to suffer. By these divisions, its body is being split and chipped away from the "Rock." This is why the Good Shepherd suffers over His wandering flock as He looks for disciples, ambassadors, priests, ministers, and shepherds. Where are my shepherds? I sought for one, but I could find none. (see Ezk. 34)

Each ministry is distinctive, having its own personality. "There is a variety of gifts but always the same Spirit; there are all sorts of service to be done, but always to the same Lord; working in all sorts of different ways in different people, it is the same God who is working in all of them." (1 Co. 12:4–6) The charismatic gifts are not usually all present in one individual. However, in a corporate ministry of believers bearing its own distinctive personality, there can be found all the gifts. Through them God supplies abundance for the welfare of the believing community.

To minister to God's people is to labor in God's name. The shepherd must labor arduously out in the fields, *getting his hands dirty.* This is the picture of the true shepherd. The Trinity (the Godhead) is at work in Him. The Father, Who is Creator of the world, redeems His creation, fallen man, through His Son, Jesus, the Good Shepherd. The Christ, in turn, continues to allow the Father and Himself to live in us through His Holy Spirit. Not being visible to us as a person, except through His creation, God the Father does become visible to us through His Son, Jesus, the Good Shepherd. Jesus, therefore, continues as the Good Shepherd to dwell among us, to nourish us, and to manifest Himself to us. This is the Holy Trinity loving us! The gifts that function through the humanity of man

are the ways Christ chooses to give Himself distinctively back to His
Church. This is one facet of His immense and infinite love for man.
Through the ministries, Jesus, the Holy Spirit, and the Father are
being imparted to the Church. Thus the body becomes nourished
and healed.

A man called to ministry does not enter into any ministry because
of his own calling, his own decision, or his own training. A man does
not enter into ministry because he decides to become a healer, a
prophet, or an evangelist, but only because God gave him life, suste-
nance, preparation, and calling for his personal surrender to the
Great Shepherd, Who allows him to shepherd the flock. "Yahweh
created me when his purpose first unfolded, before the oldest of his
works. From everlasting I was firmly set, from the beginning, before
earth came into being. The deep was not, when I was born, there
were no springs to gush with water. Before the mountains were set-
tled, before the hills, I came to birth; before he made the earth, the
countryside, or the first grains of the world's dust. When he fixed
the heavens firm, I was there, when he drew a ring on the surface of
the deep, when he thickened the clouds above, when he fixed fast
the springs of the deep, when he assigned the sea its boundaries—
and the waters will not invade the shore—when he laid down the
foundations of the earth, I was by his side, a master craftsman,
delighting him day after day, ever at play in his presence, at play everywhere in his world, delighting to be with the sons of men." (Pr.
8:22–31)

In my vocation and in my distinctive ministry of healing, it is
Christ, the Gift of Gifts, who is being given to effect the renewal of
mankind. If Christ is not personified through my sermons, my behavior, my manhood, my priesthood, my shepherding, I become
what Paul calls "a gong booming or a cymbal clashing." (1 Co.
13:1) Then would I not only fall short of being another Christ, I
would fail my commitment, my consecration to building up the
body of the Church.

To be an authentic ambassador in Christ, a docile disciple, a
truthful evangelist, and a loving shepherd means to recognize at this
very moment that God is calling all Christians to become a mighty
force sorely needed in our day. Ministers who are authentic in their
belief in charismatic renewal pose no threat to the body of Christ,
as a new movement within or parallel to the Church. Rather, they

regard their perspective within the Church as a natural part of its life, function, and expression.

Always, through many ministries, it is to the Christ that people must be led: It is to His sheepfold, in His grazing, by His nurturing that the flock is sustained. As shepherds, we are solely His bridge over which God's people walk to Him. We are His mouthpiece, through which He delivers the words of everlasting life; His feet, whose prints the struggling wanderer follows on his journey home. We are His hands, through which the Wounded Healer imposes the divine touch of healing upon the wounded seeker.

"[F]or their sake I consecrate myself so that they too may be consecrated in truth." (Jn. 17:19) Once the shepherd surrenders to the Christ, there will surge forth from his soul the Voice of Him Who called him to serve: "I shall give you your full term of life." (Ex. 23:26)

5

SPEAK MY NAME,
BE MY PRESENCE

*God has created me to do Him some definite
service: He has committed some work to me
which He has not committed to another. I
have my mission—I may never know it in
this life, but I shall be told it in the
next. . . .*

A Meditation
by CARDINAL NEWMAN

God would not be so unjust as to forget all you have done, the love
that you have for his name or the services you have done, and are
still doing, for the saints. (Heb. 6:10)

Perusing the passages of Scripture, we can readily see how God finds
ways to bring His message to His people. Love will always find a way
for communication. The Holy Word echoes forth: "He called the
Twelve together and gave them power and authority over all devils
and to cure diseases, and he sent them out to proclaim the kingdom
of God and to heal." (Lk. 9:1–2)

Each apostle is an individual. Each individual apostle is one sent forth. In being sent forth he is a messenger. The one who is sent forth is a person who is chosen. He who was chosen is one who is loved. Isaiah 43:1 confirms this concept in his reflective statement: "I have called you by name, you are mine."

In considering these thoughts, one cannot help but realize that the authors are speaking of a special commission. He who has been selected for a special commission is he who is capable of carrying out his entrustment, because he or she has been fully authorized. Endowed with such authorization, he who is commissioned is sent out as a representative of the sender. Between the two, the commissioned and the sender, there exists a bond of connection, a link as in a chain, because of the obligations and responsibilities of obedience and accountability.

Cardinal Newman, in "A Meditation," unfolds this concept further:

> I am a link in a chain, a bond of connection between persons. He has not created me to naught. I shall do His work. I shall be an angel of peace, a preacher of truth in my own place while not intending it—if I do but keep His commandments.

With reference to the Apostolate of Prayer for Healing, such a bond of accountability exists and links me to the Church. I am privileged to function in the healing phase as one of the Church's renewal processes. After long periods of scrutiny, observation, prudence, prayer, and ecclesial direction, the Church—both on the local and on the outreach apostolate—grants me the jurisdictional right and privilege to function. But my functioning in such capacity essentially represents the ministerial gifts of my ecclesial superiors. They endorse the ministry of the Lord for the welfare of God's people, the Church. Their episcopal power of apostolicity is thus an extension of the fullness of their priesthood.

Without obedience, without accountability, commission would be as insubstantial as a charlotte russe. One of the outstanding marks of both the growth and the solidity of the Catholic Church has been the apparent hard compliance among persons one to another, of subject to superior, of self-surrender to the surrender of another. This is the rock of organization. This is the bloodstream that feeds the organism of sound mind and healthy body. This is holy obedience. The Catholic Church has always flourished through obedience. It makes one successful before the eyes of God and fosters the welfare of one's contemporaries.

Obedience is not an acquired attitude or disposition. It is learned, it is assimilated, it is digested and becomes the vim, the vigor, the vitality of a truly mature man who goes through life not as a walking encyclopedia of cerebral knowledge alone but as one who has matured through character formation. This is truly the man of God— dependable and loyal, even if life's unforeseen conditions may trip him now and then along the path to which he has been called.

Obedience, for me personally, is a solid condition. In all responsibility, I could not require adherent, staunch behavior from those who work with me unless I myself had surrendered unreservedly in staunch, adherent obedience to those whom I would necessarily have to represent. Authority is very important in my life. In order for me to perform comfortably in my work of the Church—free of distraction and doubts—I need the security and assurance that flow from authoritative obedience. I find this essential to my personality.

The very person of Jesus Himself would be there to haunt me if I would be anything else. He Himself was obedient to His Father's commands, obedient unto death.

Obedience has been one of the major factors in determining the authenticity of my ministry. Obedience was the very bloodstream that flowed forth into the formation of the Apostolate of Prayer for Healing. Obedience offered growth by means of its subjection; it produced a balanced and reliable way for the welfare and benefit of the Church at large. A man without obedience is a self-centered man. He becomes a god unto himself, a god of egocentricity. God cannot use a proud man. When authority flows from its true source, God, ministry is blessed. Before exporting such a ministry for the use of the Church, my local superiors had to exercise utmost prudence and discernment; they not only recognized, but also perceived in the ministry a constant, sincere obedience. At the proper moment in time, with the appropriate gift of their office, they accepted God's expression of charism as perceived in this particular ministry.

As would be expected, difficulties did come along the way. What true vocation does not experience the alchemization and formation of a work of merit without the purifying flames and the hammering touch of a skilled forger? And so it was to be.

The hand of forging holy obedience was about to strike a chosen vessel. In so doing, a sound would be echoed forth, heard, and distinguished as to its unworth or worth. The hand of the Master was to make a giant stroke. The local superiors, bearing within themselves the fullness of the Holy Spirit's discernment, bearing within themselves the genius of the forger craftsman's skillful touch, assembled personally with me. The meeting was a simple but deliberate one. The Holy Spirit was working in unison among us. The art of Gamaliel would intervene tactfully but decisively:

> Then he addressed the Sanhedrin, "Men of Israel, be careful how you deal with these people. . . . What I suggest, therefore, is that you leave these men alone and let them go. If this enterprise, this movement of theirs, is of human origin it will break up of its own accord; but if it does in fact come from God you will not only be unable to destroy them, but you might find yourselves fighting against God." (Ac. 5:35, 38–39)

Looking directly into my eyes, my bishops expressed not only warmth, respect, and concern but also a profound insight. "We know who you are and what you have been. We know you are an obedient priest. Do you understand our position? Do you understand that our position, as well as our office, now demands us to make concise decisions? Would you be willing to close up this ministry of healing at St. Bernard's Church in Fitchburg until further discernment can be had?" I looked them in the eyes and conveyed to them the response of sincerity and respect and love that I bore for them. My reply was "Yes, Bishop, why not? If this is what you wish, then I must continue to be what you wish me to be: a true priest of Christ." At my yes, their eyes excitedly opened in relief. "You will?" "Yes, Bishop, why not? It's not my ministry that will be taking a respite. It's God's." Then, with a smile, I added: "It's rest time. I am kind of tired, anyway."

Their remarks now took the Holy Spirit's directive: "Well, then," they said, "we would like you to go away for a good period of time. Have you had your vacation yet?" I knew what was coming and with every intention to accommodate the moment, I replied: "No, I haven't, but I'm sure glad time is going to provide." With his own sense of humor my good bishop said: "Take about three or four weeks of vacation and go as far away as you can." So I decided to go to my cousin's in Florida, where the temperature in August was hotter than it was at this moment in that chancery office. I replied: "I have my three weeks' vacation coming. I can take it now, if you so wish." One of the two bishops present immediately inserted: "Take four if you want, and don't let anyone know where you are going. Relax. You need a rest. You are tired. You can sleep and rest and recuperate."

Now came the Master's final stroke of discernment. "After the vacation is completed, you will go to an enclosed retreat house; there you will spend thirty days. During those days, under the guidance of four priests, you will be observed and discerned as to the validity of the spirit and the phenomena functioning through you. Moreover, at your final service, this Thursday, at St. Bernard's Church, you will deliver an appropriate prepared speech to the thronging congregation assembled to hear you."

I smiled in amusement at what was actually transpiring here.

I realized the burden placed upon my spiritual father, my Ordinary, my bishop and my friend, who would not hurt me, but who had the welfare of the Church at heart, as well as mine. He was offering me the true sign of a follower of Christ: the practice of holy obedience.

What I believe he was doing, whether he recognized it or not, was what Christ had done with Peter before he had commissioned him for the tremendous responsibility of service and labor in the vineyard of the Lord. He was taking a little pebble, his priest, and placing it in the mixture of cement, thus to produce a cornerstone of stability and of worth.

On that following Thursday night in the middle of August 1978, I conducted the usual overflow assembly of devotees in a final farewell service of prayer for healing. At the moment of the Gospel, I approached the pulpit from whence messages of hope and love and faith so often went forth from my priestly heart. With a feeling of sadness that accompanies farewells, I raised my voice in tune with the written message of good-bye. I staunchly adhered to the prepared message, which is not my ordinary custom. But the necessity for accuracy and the necessity to prevent any misinterpretation among the people required the following:

> In the past year and some months, you have shared your concerns with me, and I have shared mine with you. It has been a wonderful

experience. The Lord has been good to you, and more than good to me.

These past months have been particularly taxing. I have told you about people asking me to go to Europe, to Hawaii, to almost every state in the union—in a word, to go all over the world. These requests have caused me to reflect prayerfully about what the Lord is asking of me as His priest, His servant.

I do not know what He wants. Like you, I have to search His will in my regard. I have to discern. Discernment implies long, deep, and even painful searching in prayer. At this point in my life, I have to pray all the longer. The Good News of Jesus uses the words: "Come apart and rest awhile." I really need that.

Like each one of you, I am human. I am body and soul. My body is tired. My soul needs nourishment. I need to go "apart."

Bishop Flanagan has granted that I be allowed to go on vacation tomorrow and then go on a long period of retreat. The Lord does not work by the clock, so I am going to give Him plenty of time.

I am setting out in faith. Only the Lord knows where I am to be led. I am putting myself completely in His hands, confident that with the guidance of His Spirit I will be led to do what He wants me to do, and whenever and wherever that might be, using my priesthood to bring people to a deeper love and knowledge of Jesus.

I hope you will understand and accept this need of mine. As always, I ask that you pray for me so I can grow in the Lord and build up the Church, the body of Christ. You can be sure that I will continue to pray for you and yours.

May God bless all of us!

So I went away and I took my vacation of four weeks. I spent much time in reading and writing, but mostly in prayer. Time was good to me, as it has always been. After my vacation, I spent thirty days in the seclusion of a seminary in Warwick, Rhode Island, under the prudent guidance, direction, and observation of a beautiful, charismatic-educated priest, Father George Kosicki, C.S.B. As I reminisce over those days I cannot help but realize that the response of my priestly obedience to legitimate authority bore much more conviction than the very acts of holistic healings. My bishop was not abandoning the Church, nor his people, and he would also respect the character of the priesthood in me. He was the shepherd. He bore the fullness of priesthood. I was just an extension of the priesthood in him, ever since the time he adopted me into his own diocese. The gifts of healing, as all the other full gifts, were really his. With all things in proper focus, priorities and so forth, he now was able with certitude to prepare me for the work of the Church. And so through the medium of holistic healings I was to fulfill one of the great activities of priestly power: to teach and preach the message of the Master. Thus, by the very essence and nature of what was taking place, a healing evangelist was being formed.

As time unfolded into months and years, and with further guidance on Church procedures and policies, I met with greater understanding and acceptance from other ecclesial superiors. These men, in turn, through their own intense life of prayer and unity with the Holy Spirit—desiring the welfare of the Church along with its growth—took moments to observe what God Himself was working, organizing, developing, evolving, shaping: all the elements that were holy and necessary for a contemporary Church in pursuit of a new Pentecost.

I am frequently asked where I see my ministry heading. My response is twofold: First, I do best where I am placed at the present moment. From a practical standpoint, I am most effective when I concentrate on the here and now. My second response flows from that which is actually occurring in this moment of my apostolate. In God's unfolding plan, I see this ministry as being epitomized by the command of Christ to go forth and to preach to all peoples: "All authority in heaven and on earth has been given to me. Go, therefore, make disciples of all the nations." (Mt. 28:18–19) Moreover, I foresee the ministry of healing as a praying apostolate, as a stepping-stone, as a shining star to evangelization.

The first apostles spent three years with Jesus during His own public ministry. They personally experienced His presence both human and divine. They knew He suffered, died, and was buried. They witnessed Him with their own senses of perception. They saw Him alive after His resurrection. On Olivet's heights they absorbed with a profound impression the message of commission. On Pentecost Sunday they emerged from the Cenacle as giants of the faith.

Empowered with the gifts of the Holy Spirit, with the supportive intercessory prayers of Mary, the mother of Jesus, they went forth into the arenas of the world to lay the foundation of His Church.

With respect to myself, I perceive more clearly at each moment of my daily prayer, especially during my daily Holy Hour, that I am being rightly used in my priesthood to continue in some degree the building up and the healing of the body of the Church. But we know and see in the world powerful influences attacking and altering God's people. The forces of good, if recognized, if complied with, become far more surpassing powers of influence. On the other hand, those of us called to the service of the people must be honest enough to recognize the onslaught of evil forces. Such dangers as pragmatism, secularism, occultism, materialism, and immorality of all sorts are attacking the body of the Church through subtle ways. God does not abandon His people. He hears the cry of the poor, of the oppressed; their tears water the very land upon which He placed them. He bends down to wipe away their tears. Their voices cry in agony for healing that surpasses the human touch. Their wounds are spiritual. Their medication is divine and their prognosis is a renewed people.

God has brought Himself to the presence of His people through external manifestations. These manifestations, or charisms, are powerful, awesome, overwhelming to the eyes of all who perceive—so much so that dazed people continue to investigate. They search, they grope to and fro. Finally, after intense pain and anguish, they suddenly and surprisingly realize that God was always in their midst. His very own Christ embraced them with His compassionate, outstretched arms. And like Hosea of the Scriptures, they did not know that He stooped down and healed them.

> When Israel was a child I loved him,
> and I called my son out of Egypt.
> But the more I called to them, the further
> they went from me; they have offered
> sacrifice to the Baals and set their offerings
> smoking before the idols.
> I myself taught Ephraim to walk,
> I took them in my arms;
> Yet they have not understood that I was the
> one looking after them.
>
> (Ho. 11:1–3)

I am like many others who carry their own charisms as personifications of Jesus Christ among His people, being uniquely used for what I consider the building on the foundations that were laid down by Jesus and His original apostles. Those who respond wholeheartedly to the Master's call for the building up of the Church are similar, I believe, to St. Francis of Assisi, who, in his time, was also uniquely used to repair the wounds of the Church. Each age supplies its own healers. Francis had been called by Christ, personally, through no human intervention. Christ said to him, "Francis, build My Church." Was he not communicating intimately with Francis? Was not the message the same: Heal My Church, which has been wounded by the attacks of satanic forces. Truly, then, God the Divine Physician sends healers to every age. If God is to remain the ever-loyal God that He is, He in turn must remedy the weaknesses that are always going to arise out of the broken humanity of His people. To reiterate, the healer's task is to apply the Divinity of Christ, Who is the head of the Church, to the diseases and infected cells of His mystical body.

What was Jesus' aim in calling the twelve apostles? What is Jesus' aim in calling our bishops? What is Jesus' aim in calling John Paul II? What is Jesus' aim in calling ministers and priests? What is Jesus' aim in calling me? What is Jesus' aim in calling us? We see in Mark 3:14 that He ordained twelve that they should be with him, identify with Him. He sent them out to preach. Through their preaching, He Himself continued to teach, minister, and heal. That they should have experience of His presence was tremendously important to their calling: "It is you who have stood by me through my trials." "If any man will open the door, I will come in." And so He allows us to open the door for His life, and that very same act, I believe, is what He is doing through us, through me. He is opening the door to all the facets of our lives, coalescing them into oneness, purifying them, giving them purpose.

With each one of us—our filtered, purified selves—He utilizes our life's homespun experiences, our education, our training, to give Himself as gift.

God respects the processes of human psychology. He endowed us with this functional gift. So, too, in order to allow Himself to be experienced by man, He uses visible signs and wonders to bring us to the knowledge of Himself. Without this method of visible signs disclosing the invisible, we finite human beings are unable to grasp the invisible life of God.

As human beings, we must hear something, see something, touch something, taste something, experience the presence of reality. God knows this, and through external manifestations, therefore, He awakens man to the presence of His power. God's tool is the manifestation of His Spirit.

Those who wish to become ambassadors of God, being convinced of His power by experimental observation or theoretical argument, conclude: I want to be like him. I want God in my life. What is happening here is that God is drawing them to Himself as He did with the apostles. He is causing them to admire Him, and then He is drawing them from admiration into His love. This is the spiritual psychology of the loving divine heart.

Jesus, with all His might, wanted His apostles to love Him. Utilizing new signs and wonders, He drew them unto Himself. They ended up as friends of His love. Jesus became their alpha and their omega. Then, too, even the human nature of Jesus wanted their sympathy. How often they saw Jesus tired and hungry in His humanity. We who follow the Christ must also recognize with open eyes, we must also hear with truly open ears, the cries of the broken Christ that are seen in His poor ones and His own suffering. Although Jesus, the Christ, can no longer suffer, because He is a resurrected and ascended God dwelling in the glory of heaven, He nevertheless continues to suffer in time in His broken body, the Church, His people. This is what Jesus said to Saul when He converted him. There, upon that ground on the road to Damascus, Saul, slain in the spirit, hears the voice of Jesus of Nazareth: "Saul, Saul, why are you persecuting me?" "Who are you, Lord?" he asked? And the voice came forth like a piercing spear, sharp and to the point: "I am Jesus of Nazareth, whom you are persecuting." And Saul, astounded, convicted unto the truth, simulated innocence as he said: "I do not persecute you. I persecute Christians."

There it was in that very response that Saul convicted himself of his own crime. Truth would have its vindication. Justice would have its restoration, and Jesus as both prosecuting attorney and judge replied that the Christians whom Saul was persecuting belonged to Him.

Christ must live in the apostles; and He Who called them as chosen vessels for ambassadorship must reign in them. The genuine call to be a valid ambassador of God, therefore, derives from THE CHRIST (the Christ is the primary cause of ministering). The one chosen to be the instrument of ambassadorship is he who becomes the instrument of the Christ. The Holy Spirit is the agent working through the ambassador who brings about the salvation of the soul and its sanctification.

What is this Church that you and I are called to serve? What is this Church that you and I are vocationally obligated to represent in this modern age? It is the same Church that John Paul II so gallantly sustains on the shoulders of his consecrated humanity . . . it is the same Church that received the precious blood of Jesus as He was hanging upon the Cross . . . it is the same Church that was enriched and further nourished in imitation of its Master and Founder by the blood of the martyrs . . . it is the same Church to which ministers and priests and men of true dedication to the causes of God are summoned. It is the Church that serves the body of Christ in all men.

> Keep Jesus Christ in your hearts and you will recognize His face in every human being. You will want to help Him out in all His needs: the needs of your brothers and sisters. (John Paul II)

Christ has no hands but our hands to do His work today; He has no feet but our feet to lead men in their way; He has no tongue but our tongue to tell men how He died; He has no help but our help to bring them to decide for Him.

Does the Master's call relate to us? We are His disciples and we can share in being His apostles, for one cannot be a true disciple who is not prepared to be an apostle. Christ counts on each of us. He counts on every individual. He plays no games with mankind.

Nineteen hundred years ago, Christ counted on a group of young people to change the world. So, too, today He counts on us, young and old, men and women, to decide to follow Him. His call to us is sudden, abrupt, final. The English painter William Holman (1827–1910), in his masterpiece, "The Light of the World," depicts Christ knocking at the door at night. The door does not have a latch on the outside, and Jesus comes to knock only once as He passes by. That door can be opened only from the inside.

But before that hour of decision, when Jesus knocks on the door, the genuinely called apostle has had an intimate acquaintance with Jesus. From my infancy onward, I experienced companionship with Jesus. It prepared the way. As a little boy, my mother's closeness to the Church, my admiration for the holy parish priest for whom I served eight years as altar boy, the experiences I had with him that kept feeding me the holiness of Jesus Christ, all were aspects of my developing companionship with Christ. For me, the parish priest was truly Jesus Christ on earth. I loved him. I esteemed the priesthood that he bore so conscientiously, even scrupulously. As I look back, I see that, by God's Divine Providence, I was especially blessed to walk from my mother's arms to the embrace of the Roman Catholic Church by walking always in the company of Jesus.

Besides companionship with Jesus, another necessary quality for apostleship is simplicity. Although distinctively blessed, a man must bc in his own heart simple. He must be a humble friend of Jesus. Jesus is most comfortable with humble friends.

Still another important step to apostleship is detachment. Detachment in the spiritual sense means that we are severed from ourselves so that we may be attached to Christ. Such detachment often implies the sundering of home and family ties and the relinquishing of ordinary occupations and monetary gain.

That's the apostleship to which I and my brother priests have been called. Could it not also be the witnessing of the Lord to which you, our reader, may be called? Are not the words of the great nineteenth-century French philosopher-priest Lacordaire most fitting to a true ambassador?

> To live in the midst of the world with no desire for its pleasures; to be a member of every family, yet belong to none; to share all sufferings, all joys, to penetrate all secrets; to heal all wounds; to go daily from men to God; to offer Him their homage and petition; to return from God to men to bring them His pardon and His hope; to have a heart of bronze for chastity; to teach and instruct; to pardon and console; to bless and be blessed forever! What a wonderful life! And it is yours, O PRIEST OF JESUS CHRIST!

Though the call may be hard and strenuous, God sustains with ample grace. The apostles themselves gave up their fishermen's nets. They gave up the tax collector's bench. They followed The Lord in a moment of decision. The Master's call to apostleship wants the whole of us, all of us, just as we are, with all our sins, all our sorrows, all our joys. That's why He died. His dying voice from the tree of life continues ever onward in its echo: "Give me your sins. I will wash you clean in My blood. You are Mine. I have called you by name. Allow Me to embrace you. Allow Me to love you. Take Me down from this cross, that My arms may fall around you in a holy embrace."

On the natural level, the ambassador is an envoy, the officially appointed representative of one government in the territory of another government. In the spiritual order, he represents heaven's government on earth. Being ambassadors in Christ, called to the evangelistic mission, requires that we clarify to clergy and laity alike that they recognize all Christians within the Church as a mighty force. Generous souls are needed in our day in a special way for the strengthening and building up of the Church. Our ambassadorship should not offer a threat to the body of Christ as though we were a new movement with, or parallel to, the Church. Whatever gifts we have are used to place evangelism within the framework of the Church as a natural part of its life and function and expression. Evangelism is the tool of the ambassador. When we preach the message of salvation, we express ambassadorship through evangelism. Our primary concern is not to preach a "good sermon" but, rather, to kindle and strengthen faith in God through the work of the Holy Spirit. Evangelism, therefore, is the tool of the healing ministry. To be an authentic evangelist is to be an authentic ambassador. To deliver the message of God, the Good News, implies that, through the Word, men may be confronted in a very personal way with the Christ the Word represents.

With St. Paul (Ep. 6:18–20) we say: "Pray all the time, asking for what you need, praying in the Spirit on every possible occasion. Never get tired of staying awake to pray for all the saints; and pray for me to be given an opportunity to open my mouth and speak without fear and give out the mystery of the gospel of which I am an ambassador in chains; pray that in proclaiming it I may speak as boldly as I ought to."

> Therefore, I will trust Him. Whatever, wherever, I am. I can never be thrown away. If I am in sickness, my sickness may serve Him: In perplexity, my perplexity may serve Him: If I am in sorrow, my sorrow may serve Him. He does nothing in vain. He knows what He is about. He may take away my friends, He may throw me among strangers, He may make me feel desolate, make my spirits sink, hide my future from me—still He knows what He is about.

> A MEDITATION
> CARDINAL NEWMAN

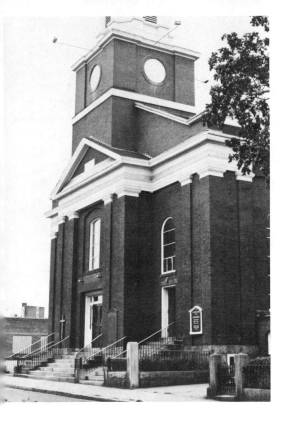

*St. John's Church
(Worcester, Massachusetts)*

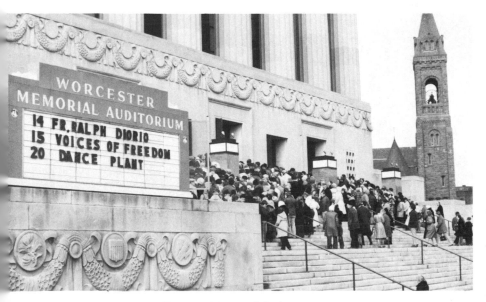

Worcester Memorial Auditorium

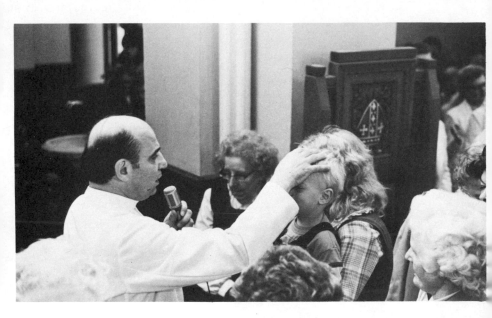

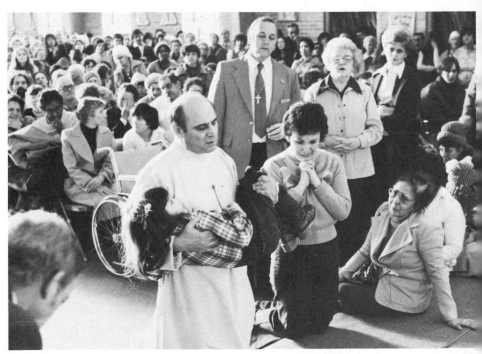

"Let the children come to me."

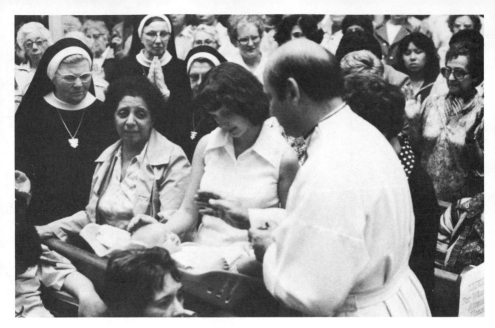

After anointing a baby with holy oil

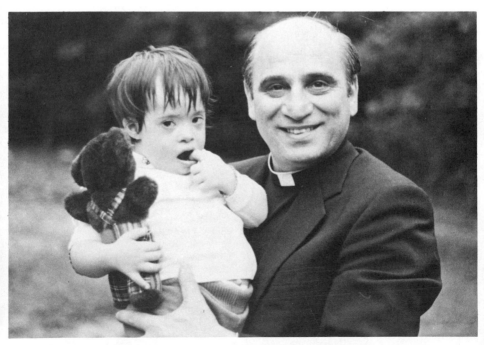

Young Sarah deMoon, thought to be suffering from Down's syndrome, after healing of severe facial deformities

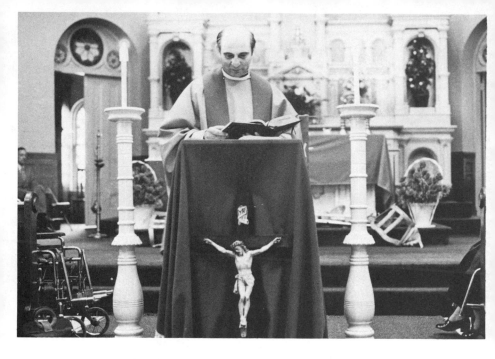

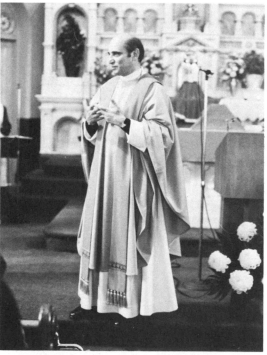

Preaching the written word of evangelization

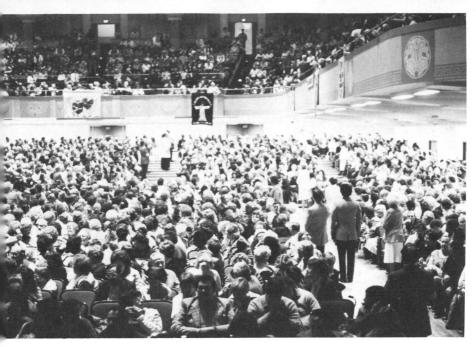

Going among the crowd to give personal blessings

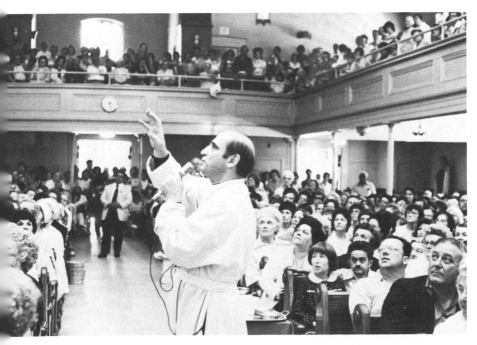

Father uses the gift of knowledge to call out healings.

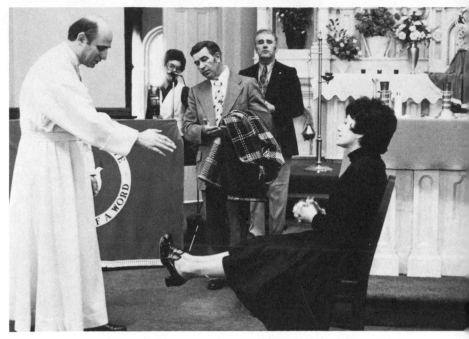

A short leg grows.

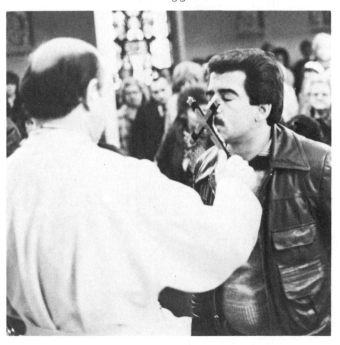

The power of the Cross—a kiss of love

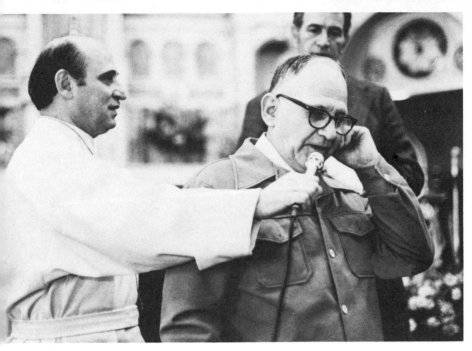

The deaf hear . . .

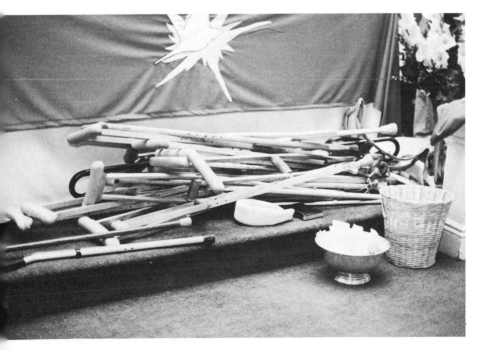

. . . and the lame walk.

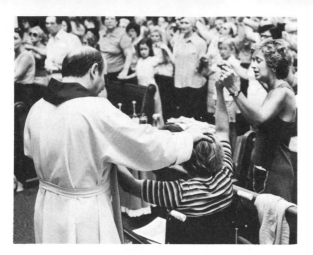
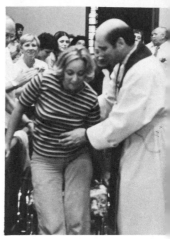

The power of laying on of hands

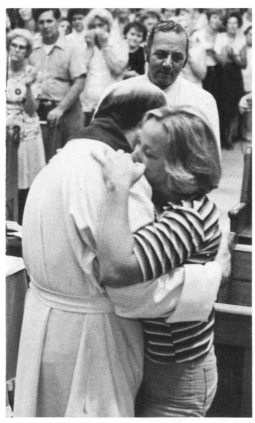

Gratitude for intercessory prayers after receiving a healing

6

I HEARD HIS VOICE
AND COULD ONLY SAY "YES"

The Lord will always call,
and there will always be responses
on the part of people who are ready and willing.
He needs, and He wants to need,
your person, your intelligence, your energy,
your faith, your love, your holiness.
He wants to speak to the people of today
through your voice.
He wants to consecrate the Eucharist
and forgive sins through you.
He wants to love with your heart.
He wants to help with your hands.
He wants to save through your efforts.
Think about it carefully;
the response that many of you can give
is given personally to Christ,
Who is calling you to these great things.

POPE JOHN PAUL II

If God calls us, if He invites us to follow in a given way, He does so in order that we may respond with our own lives to the gift we have received from Him. The Christian must always, and in all circumstances, be able to repeat, with faith and with conviction, the words of the young Samuel: "Speak, Lord, your servant is listening." (1 S. 3:9) The challenging call of Christ "Come after Me: I will make you fishers of men" will always urge the immediate abandonment of one's nets to become His followers. (Mk. 1:18 NAB)

Does the world hear His voice too? His first apostles heard His voice: "Come follow Me." "Peter was moved to say to Him: 'We have put aside everything to follow You!' Jesus answered: 'I give you My word, there is no one who has given up home, brothers or sisters, mother or father, children or property, for Me and for the gospel who will not receive in this present age *a hundred times as many homes, brothers and sisters, mothers and fathers, children and property—and persecution besides—and in the age to come, everlasting life.'*" (Mk. 10:28–30 NAB)

One who so answers the Christ is one who believes and trusts the Christ. And who is more trustworthy than the Christ? To follow the Christ requires love. But who is more deserving of love than Christ, the Saviour? To follow the Master requires sacrifice, but so does everything else that is worthwhile. Answering the call of Christ to faith, trust, love, and sacrifice requires an exchange between two beings. In such a union of beings, heart speaks to heart: "*cor loquitur ad cor.*" Then love's intimacy begets the grace of sharing. Happiness must be spread and there is no greater joy than possessing Jesus and diffusing His Word. By answering the call of Christ, one in union with Christ can reach out to mankind with the Good News of salvation. And that Good News will reveal the Christ as the Way, the Truth, and the Life.

Nothing gives us greater inspiration than the example of one totally dedicated to the Lord, one who truly burns out and is burned for the sake of the God above.

From whence does a frail human being derive such strength? From whence does a vocational calling spring? From whence does the inexhaustible power continue to flow with an ever-increasing output? In what great heart of life does the human heart, the human person—tired in his humanity, yet not tired in his calling—sustain himself? This answer simply is founded between the generous heart of God and the great heart of man who is thus called. Herein two precious beings, Creator and creature, come into harmony. One knows who one is, where one is going, and Who one's God is.

Our own natural human answer to these questions lies in our willingness to share the burden of our brothers in Christ. The healing apostolate of prayer for the sick is only one instance; there are thousands of others! Every man, woman, and child is called. Every man, woman, and child is chosen. We are life for one another.

John Paul II exhorts all mankind to "give your life with joy." In so doing, one is brought into the requiem of Silent Prayer, into a personal interlude of a voyage of self-revelation, into a tenebrae of darkness in order to see the light of a new horizon. In so praying, God's call will be a crystallization of one's vocation. In so hearing the call, the recipient must respond as he or she unravels all the experiences of time, circumstances, events, thus harmonizing them into a wholeness of a true vocation. Yes, two hearts have come into communication: God has spoken; man has heard. "*Cor loquitur ad cor*," as so well described by St. Augustine.

Some persons respond negatively both to life and to their God. Others respond with positiveness. Some great souls answer their call with tremendous responsibility, fear, and trembling. But *respond* one must, if one is truly to find the purpose of his existence. Whether or not one responds to the divine call to serve, the Creator of life loves His people. And like a "Hound of Heaven" He will search and probe and sensitize the human soul into a response. In so seeking the human soul's response, the Author of life is attempting to extend His presence among men. He does this through many forms: Creator, Provider, Healer, Restorer. Because God will not leave His children on earth as orphans, His call will be constant. Yes, the Lord will always call. And there will always be responses on the part of many people who are ready and willing.

A call to serve the Lord comes to every person, both in the religious life and in the secular. Like the boy Samuel, whom God had repeatedly called, so in my own young life I, too, responded to the call of the Lord: "Here I am (O Lord), since You called me"— *Ecce ego (Domine): quia vocasti me.* "Behold, I come to do Your will, O God"—*Ecce venio, ut faciam, Deus, voluntatem tuam.* (see 1 Sam. 3:6 and Heb. 10:9)

My intention to become a priest seeded itself with particular influence from my mother's family. Her family ties gave many vocations to the service of God, one including, as I am told, a prelate. Such roots and seed were nurtured in and at my home through prayer, work, sacrifice, and much suffering. At the age of eight, following my First Holy Communion, the local parish priests under the direction of the Missionary Fathers of St. Charles, otherwise known as the Scalabrini Priests, perpetuating the name of Bishop John Baptist Scalabrini, their founder, took a deep personal interest in my life. Through their influence and direction I entered their seminary program. Although, at fifteen years of age, in the autumn of 1945, I entered the Sacred Heart Minor Seminary, in Melrose Park, Illinois, under the auspices and educational discipline of this religious congregation of priests and lay brothers for Italian immigrants, that entrance, as I look back, now seems to me to have been the outward sign of a choice that had been made long before by a Divine Providence. God had called. My response was "Yes."

For twelve long years my spirit and soul and body unfolded in strict discipline, study, piety. Every successful priest must have his foundation in these elements. Every successful priest must fly on two wings: one of knowledge and one of holiness. Both these endeavors became my constant concern and successful achievement. On Saturday morning, June 1, 1957, at 9:17 A.M., twelve long, intensive years having been completed since entering the seminary, I was ordained a priest of Jesus Christ through the imposition of hands of Bishop Raymond J. Hillinger, D.D., Auxiliary Bishop of Chicago. On that a day a thousand and one thoughts coursed through my mind. I stood in wonderment at God's power to raise men of all sorts to be his ambassadors. The words of Pius XI came to me with exceptional force:

> And now, finally, to you dear Children, Priests of the Most High, both secular and regular, the world over, We address Our words. You are "Our glory and joy," you, who with such great generosity bear the "burden of the day and the heat," you, who so powerfully help Us and Our Brethren of the Episcopate in fulfilling the duty of feeding the flock of Christ. To you We send Our Paternal thanks and Our warmest encouragement. We know and fully appreciate your admirable zeal; and to it, in the needs of the present, We make this heartfelt appeal. These needs are becoming daily graver.

All the more must your redeeming work grow and intensify; for "you are the salt of the earth, and the light of the world."*

I looked around at the other newly ordained priests. On ordination day the new priest dedicates his entire life to the work God has chosen for him alone to do. For some this would mean a lifetime of prayer, their heads hidden beneath a cowl. For others it would mean working quietly, unobtrusively, behind a desk. Still others would be leaving home for the frozen wastes of the Far North, for jungles and swamps, for the stricken neighborhoods of the poor, the sick, and the suffering. They would serve in large cities, in villages, and in towns. How true: The whole world is a priest's parish.

When the Holy Spirit had completed His mysterious work in the souls of my classmates Vince, Chuck, Eddie, and Michael (now deceased), and myself, I was then clothed in the vestments of my office. God Himself imbued the spirit of His priesthood into my soul through the Bishop's hands. The long-expected day had dawned at last. The distant vision and boyhood dreams of long ago now suddenly brightened and cheered my ascension to the summit of the holy throne of a priest's glory, the *Roman Catholic Priesthood*. The day had come which God had appointed for me from all eternity! Only men as followers of a Leader so great as Christ can fathom the profundity of the indelible scar upon our souls: *"Tu est sacerdos in aeternum"*—Thou art a priest forever!

It was for this precise day that men like myself were created, that the early years of our lives were surrounded with special care and attention by a kind and wise Divine Provider. It was precisely for this day of ordination that God had entrusted to His priests the delicate and arduous work of Christian evangelization. Only a priest, on the day of his ordination, as he kneels before the august presence, in the brokenness and weakness and nothingness of his humanity, can suddenly realize all his prayers, all his labors, all his struggles, as being crowned by the great High Priest, Jesus Christ. A great transformation takes place in the soul and character of such a one called to the priesthood, an indelible mark to remain throughout time and eternity. Along with my classmates, I had become God's representative among men, an ambassador of Christ, partaker of His power, dispenser of His grace and merits, keeper of His sacred

* Encyclical on the Catholic priesthood.

revealed mysteries, leader of a people exiled through an exodus of human barrenness and human trial, successor of all the holy priests who for many centuries have continued Christ's mission to the world.

And so, for the eighth and last time since the day of my tonsure, I gladly answered the archdeacon's call, the most momentous of all: "Here I am, O Lord, I am ready to accept the obligations of the priesthood as well as its high dignity, its beauties as well as its rights, its responsibilities as well as its powers. I willingly offer myself to You, soul and body, to spend the rest of my life and to be spent for the noble work which You shall entrust to me through Your holy Church. *Adsum!*"

And so the time had come when the great miracle was to be performed in my soul. Bishop Hillinger and the priests present, one by one, solemnly imposed their hands upon my classmates and upon myself. Thus they imparted to us the character, power, and grace of the priesthood, of which they are the depositaries. They called down upon us the heavenly gifts, the blessings of the Holy Spirit, and the strength of priestly grace. The dream of my youth had been realized.

My own experience in the priesthood has ranged widely. My first assignment after ordination was as a summer replacement at St. Michael's, on the West Side of Chicago. Most of the people in the parish were from Tuscany, in northern Italy. They had come to America after World War II, and many were little better off than they had been in war-devastated Italy. A number of them were outspoken Communists. I learned in St. Michael's parish that no one is beyond the reach of God's outstretched hand.

My next assignment was as second assistant pastor in the Santa Maria Addolorata parish, on the South Side of Chicago. There, under Father Alex Peloso, the pastor, I learned that the practical aspects of life should not be ignored, that the road to higher understanding would sometimes open up only when approached through tending to the day-by-day concerns and desires of our parishioners. I became involved in a number of youth programs and discovered that there were great ministerial benefits in working with young people.

Throughout the early years of my priesthood I was assigned varied ministerial duties. Many of these duties were in the fields of pastoral care; others were in teaching, lecturing, hospital, retreat, radio, and youth work. Whatever parish or assignment I was given, each change served as another stepping-stone, another piece of the mosaic of the future "man beneath the gift."

During one of my assignments, a serious illness had befallen me which had its roots in seminary days. The illness itself was another formative experience along this unfolding road that God was mapping out for me.

To lighten my load, while I slowly recovered my strength, I was assigned to Mother Cabrini parish, in Chicago, the parish where I had been ordained. In conjunction with parochial duties I also taught and lectured, conducted youth retreats and parish renewal weekends, and served as hospital chaplain to the sick. I loved all these ministries immensely. Then, in order to satisfy the influx of a Hispanic immigration, I also attended Spanish classes under the auspices of the diocesan Chicago Apostolate.

"Where was God calling me?" It was while serving in Mother Cabrini parish that I began to ask that question. I wondered whether the road I was traveling as a Scalabrinian Priest, being solely consumed for Italian immigrants, was the right road for a priest ordained for all mankind. This thought agonized my zealous heart. I felt more and more that if I would remain with the good Scalabrinian Fathers, my full contribution, not yet completely focused, might be impaired as I tried to serve the Church in its entirety. Long periods of doubt, prayer, reflection, and anguish were resolved through objective counsel and spiritual direction from my confessors and spiritual directors. In conscience I felt a moral obligation. A resolve had to be made. I must step out in faith and follow the unknown road that would lead to "being" and not merely "achieving."

Such a change is not easily made. The wheels for exclaustration from a religious, sociological congregation move slowly, but there was forward movement in the direction I desired. However, as an intermittent step in the process of further reflection and evaluation, my superiors—in all fairness to them and to my desire—postponed my release by assigning me to the outskirts of a mining town, Atikokan, in Ontario, Canada. Again, man's interruptions became God's invitations. Among my ministerial duties of parish work and high school teaching and other educational programs in that diocese, I was privileged beyond expectation and greatly overjoyed to become friends with Protestant clergymen. So often, time would find us together working hand in hand, side by side, praying together, smiling together, suffering together, working for a common goal: *that Jesus Christ be Lord!* With such a conjunction of labor the community of Atikokan became enriched with the presence of God, the salvation of Christ, and the sanctification of the Holy Spirit. At that time, ecumenism had scarcely been heard of. Later, the concept played an important part in the development and ministry of the healing apostolate of prayer, evangelism, crusades, and programs of renewal.

In the fifth year of my priesthood, the Canadian assignment at an end, I was selected to report to the Immaculate Conception Novitiate, in Cornwall, New York, to become assistant novice master. In Cornwall, besides my teaching duties I had the great satisfaction once again to work side by side with the local Protestant ministers and the local Catholic priests. Pope John XXIII, under the inspiration of the Holy Spirit, had proclaimed to the world: "Let there be a new Pentecost where men and women of all denominations will no longer emphasize their differences, but reflect upon their identities." Like many of my fellow priests, I was fired by a new energy at this chance to reach out to all humanity with the strength of Christian unity compelling us.

The large possibilities opened by the spirit of ecumenism confirmed me in my desire to terminate finally my association with the Scalabrini Missionary Congregation. I sought to become a diocesan priest. Due to the concern of those in authority over me to lose one of their priests and thereby establish precedence for other priests who were reflecting in the same vein that I was, five more years were to pass before deciding my request. Finally, with God's grace and with the help of diocesan clergy as well as the Apostolic Delegate of Washington, D.C., permission was granted me to seek the new horizons of my priesthood. On July 1, 1967, I returned to my home, in Providence, Rhode Island, until the proper authoritative procedures were complete. During that period of time, soon after my return, my father died at the age of fifty-five. He was buried on my birthday, July 19, 1967.

Those days of arduous waiting sustained by a deep life of prayer, perseverance, and patience, were a time of crucial testing. But finally, we find His pathways. I received official notification from Rome that I was released from my vow of obedience and affiliation to the Missionary Fathers of St. Charles. And so, in March 1968, after eleven years as a Scalabrini Missionary Priest, I entered the Diocese of Worcester, Massachusetts. I was willingly accepted, according to canonical procedures, by the kind, gentle, prudent, and wise Bishop Bernard J. Flanagan, D.D.

My years in the Worcester Diocese have flourished with various assignments, fulfilling all my expectations as a diocesan priest. It was in 1972 that the final piece of the mosaic to my call was put in place. Because I knew Spanish, I was assigned to further studies and work with the growing Spanish-American community. Because of the Hispanic need for adequate pastoral attention, I was urged by my Hispanic community to expose myself to and become acquainted with the Charismatic Renewal. Under the direction and guidance of my Auxiliary Bishop, Timothy J. Harrington, I attended charismatic services for the first time. I was impressed with "old moods and new labels." The soul of the Church bore no dichotomy in this expression of union with God. The people were hungry, the people were being fed, the people sought hope in an absolute and unchangeable God. The world had betrayed: The world had made promises to people which it had not kept. Regardless of my traditional background, I had to submit my priestly expression for the good of God's people, and not my own. Was not my priesthood given to me for the building up of the Church? And so, on May 9, 1976, Mother's Day, while assisting at a charismatic service in Cambridge, Massachusetts, I openly and publicly boomed into the charism of the healing gifts.

In the months that followed, through many healing services, God clarified, through suffering and perseverance, that He had decided to use me as a conduit for His healing grace. The end of the winding road He had led me along suddenly became crystal clear, the Exodus experience had come to fruition. My priesthood, with the substance of its blessings transmitted to me, suddenly was renewed *in the power of the Holy Spirit*. I was no longer my own. God had prepared me, through the schooling of prayer, suffering, perseverance, and patience, for the splendid gift of healing evangelism. God gave me a gift. God gave me a call. I HEARD HIS VOICE, AND COULD SAY ONLY YES.

7

THE PRIEST AS GIFT

My dear sons, who are about to be consecrated to the office of the priesthood, endeavor to receive that office worthily, and once ordained, strive to discharge it in a praiseworthy manner. A priest's duties are to offer sacrifice, to bless, to govern, to preach, to baptize. (Sacerdos, etenim oportet offere, benedicere, praeesse, praedicare, et baptizare.)

from the
ROMAN ORDINATION RITE

People must think of us as Christ's servants, stewards entrusted with the mysteries of God. (1 Co. 4:1)

I am a priest forever, according to the Lord Jesus Christ. You are a priest forever, according to the Lord Jesus Christ. Together, you and I are priests forever, both in time and in eternity. "The Lord has sworn he will not repent: 'You are a priest forever according to the order of Melchizedek.'" How beautiful and impressive that day of or-

dination was, when God anointed us with the power of the Holy
Spirit. On that special day, you and I were chosen from among men
to act on behalf of men. The Church has always preserved and protected its primary service, the holy priesthood of Jesus.

Throughout the pages of history, there have been countless attacks against those who have followed zealously in the footprints of
the High Priest and Galilean, Jesus Christ. With the spirit of conviction to the teachings of Jesus, with the spirit of courage in following and walking in the pathways of Jesus, in combat and trial,
through schism and heresy, through personal struggles, the Church
of Christ, living staunchly in the hearts of its priests, has produced
the crown and glory of martyrs, confessors, doctors, and missionaries.
Satan attempts unceasingly to demolish the very heartbeat of the
transmitting love of Jesus by annihilating weak, human men endowed by God's choice alone to be the channels of His grace
through the holy priesthood.

The attacks upon the priesthood flow from within the man beneath the priest as well as from outside forces. If the priest can be
destroyed, either from within or from without, the tragedy falls
upon a people starved and abandoned by their so-called shepherds.
This tragedy is truly irreparable. Cardinal Emmanuel Suhard once
underlined, I believe, the essential conflict of a man beneath the gift
of priesthood. Every other problem and situation that a priest suffers
is only a symptom, and not the real cause, of a self-identity and
priestly crisis. Cardinal Suhard poignantly states in his book *Priests
Among Men:* "It follows as a logical consequence of our prevalent
atheism that our age has secularized, naturalized, and humanized
the priest. If we are to find the true meaning of God again, we
must rediscover the meaning of the priesthood; there will be no
return to God without a return to the priest."

The Second Vatican Council, like councils of old, has deepened
even more so the idea of the priesthood. It identifies the priest "by
the sacred power that he has . . . in the person of Christ" (*in per-
sona Christi*). Conscious of this reality, we cannot help but understand how our priesthood is "hierarchical," that is to say connected
with the power of forming and governing the priestly people (Dogmatic Constitution *Lumen Gentium* 10).

Each priest, validly ordained, takes his origin from the combination of the mission and office of Jesus Christ, our Teacher, our

Prophet, our Priest, our King. Jesus, through the power of ordination, extends His person into us through His Holy Spirit. Inspired and endowed with this power, we are sent to witness to Him in a special way in the Church and before the world.

> The priesthood in which we share through the sacrament of Orders, which has been forever "imprinted" on our souls through a special sign from God, that is to say the "character," remains in explicit relationship with the common priesthood of the faithful, that is to say the priesthood of all the baptized, but at the same time it differs from that priesthood "essentially and not only in degree." In this way the words of the author of the Letter to the Hebrews about the priest, who has been "chosen from among men . . . appointed to act on behalf of men," take on their full meaning. (Dogmatic Constitution *Lumen Gentium* 40)

Jesus has shared His priesthood with us for no other reason but to extend Himself visibly and continuously throughout time for the building up of His people, the Church. Precisely because of this implication, the priesthood calls for and demands a very particular integrity of life, an integrity that must usher itself into service. This integrity is precisely and supremely fitting for the priestly identity.

In spite of the countless strikes against the bark of Peter in which we sail, Christ Himself appears and remains as the guiding light—strengthening and beckoning us onward with our cargo of humanity. We find encouragement in the words of Exodus 19:4-6: "You yourselves have seen . . . how I carried you on eagles' wings and brought you to myself. From this you know that now, if you obey my voice and hold fast to my covenant, you of all the nations shall be my very own, for all the earth is mine. I will count you a kingdom of priests, a consecrated nation."

The Christ who calls each one of us has not left us orphans. Throughout the night, He remains our vigilant sentry, throughout the day He remains our guiding light. Jesus encouraged His followers, if you recall, when He assured that no follower of His would walk in darkness; His followers would possess the light of life. Before Jesus was taken up to heaven He gathered His disciples around Him, and He explained to them once more the meaning of his mission of salvation: "So you see how it is written that the Christ would suffer and on the third day rise from the dead, and that, in his name, repentance for the forgiveness of sins would be preached to all the nations. . . ." (Lk. 24:46–47)

It was at this precise moment, in which Jesus took leave of His apostles, that He commanded them, and through them the whole Church, each one of us, to go out and bring the message of redemption to all nations. St. Paul himself expresses this command with force in his Second Letter to the Corinthians: ". . . and he has entrusted to us the news that they are reconciled. So we are ambassadors for Christ; it is as though God were appealing through us. . . ." (2 Co. 5:19–20)

A self-identity crisis is very difficult when men like us are called to the dignity and work of the priesthood. If our own identity is assumed by Him, the High Priest, then we who become one with Him realize that we are priests in order to aim consistently and perseveringly at becoming another Christ. With Christ Jesus as Lord of our lives, He, Himself, will reign supremely in both our private lives and in our public ministerial duties. In praxis, this reality signifies that as a priest of Jesus it is no longer you or I who operates, but under His anointing—both in sanctuary and on the street, in meeting both friends and foes—it is the Christ existing and going through our lives. The priest, the *alter Christus*, alive with Christ, meets sinners and saints; he encounters all personages of life regardless of their status. As he deals with his people, permeated with Christ's being, he constantly attempts to act and treat people as Christ would.

St. Frances Cabrini, like many other saints, would often quote the thoughts of St. Paul: "I can do all things in Him who strengthens me." And so it is the man with the gift of priesthood, who, in order to sustain his priesthood and his calling, must find Christ as his strength. Christ is his special friend. Christ is his source and fountainhead. Christ is his priestly life. Each day, the man with the gift of the priesthood and the Christ with the gift in the priesthood must enter, second by second, the inner sanctum of their perennial relationship. If the man with the gift of priesthood is to be realistically efficient as an ambassador of Christ, the High Priest, then the priest's main concern is that he maintain unbreakable contact with this unfailing source of life. As a vine nourishing the branch, so Jesus' admonition to the man he has blessed with the gift of priesthood makes so much sense: "Remain in my love." (Jn. 15:9)

The story of our footsteps to the priesthood, as well as the story of
the years of our priesthood unveiled in time and in memory, are stories worth reliving. Retracing them can offer us tremendous incen-
tives to respond to His ever revitalizing invitation "Come, follow
Me." Whatever we have made of ourselves, wherever we may be,
the inevitable fact remains: We are priests of Jesus Christ; we are
priests forever. Being priests, we are called to battle. As a brother
priest, I presume nothing beyond that which God has made me.
Like you, I am a man called to the gift of priesthood. Like you, I
have been ordained a priest forever. Like you, I am called to be one
with Christ and to represent His person in time and unto eternity.
Together, we become the bulwark of God's legionnaires. Together
we encourage ourselves. Together we strengthen ourselves. Together
we walk and work for our Leader, Jesus Christ, promoting His cause,
consuming our lives for His purpose, and if it be so, nourishing the
Church with the shedding of our own blood. This is a call to victory: namely, the conquest of virtue over vice, Christ over Satan.

We are human vessels of clay for the powers that are divine. And
for this reason it is good for brother priests to speak publicly and encouragingly of one another and to one another, that the Church at
large may know that they should pray for their priests. With your
thoughts, with your humanity, with your priestly experiences, I become one with you. May I be the conscience that feels the deep
need to speak both to you and to myself, to all of us without exception—priests, both diocesan and religious, who by the virtue of the
sacrament of Holy Orders are all made brothers. Together, we express our faith in the vocation to which Christ called us, as we are
united to our legitimate bishops. With them, we serve in privilege,
sharing their special communion of sacrament and ministry. The
Mystical Body of Christ is truly built upon this foundation. As
priests, as disciples, as ambassadors, as men gifted with the person of
Christ in our lives, we are called to battle. And battle we must.

By the power of ordination a man called by Christ becomes a
priest of God, a personification of Christ, a defender of the faith.
There have been wars since the beginning of mankind, especially in
causes of truth. All wars have ended either in victory or defeat. Yet
there is one war in particular, a spiritual war, that has never come to
an end. The clash is between Satan—deceiver, liar, and fallen angel
—and God, Truth, Creator, ever supreme. The victim is man se-

duced by Satan; the redemptive Victor is Christ, sent by God the Father. Today the devil's army may appear stronger than usual. But, out of each age, God has drawn forth, called, and equipped His cause with His special soldiers. He enlists priests to fight the forces of evil. Today, more than ever before, Christ needs His soldiers. The crusade against the crimes of Lucifer is of utmost urgency.

Throughout the ages of Christianity, throughout the length and breadth of the continents, Christ, through His bishops, has consecrated many new priests. In all parts of the world there are generous men who have accepted the gift of priesthood, men from all ranks of life. They have gone into the arena of battle with the standards and armaments of Christ, with His precious blood and His most sacred Cross, with His gospel, with His Word, with his sacraments. Some great souls, whether known or not in the public eye, are true giants in the heart and mind of God, Who sees and watches over His chosen, anointed ones. They are scattered throughout the world, in jungles and in swamps, on islands and in continents, in cities and suburbs, in schools, hospitals, byways, pathways of all sorts. Some labor in the fields of administration, others teach and preach. Wherever they may be, however they may live their call, it is nevertheless the Christ living in them that breathes and palpitates the heartbeat of the Mystical Body. They have been sent as ambassadors of Christ. In the final analysis, they have been sent to teach all nations; to bring others into the fold, to be the salt of the earth, to comfort and to heal.

We priests are the visible instrument, the visible sign, the extension of the person of Christ to a wounded and broken humanity. The truth of the reality for those who have been called to the gift of priesthood is that they have become priests unreserved in their commitment. Yes, they—you and I—are priests always. No matter what circumstances or conditions prevail or encircle the time in which we live, we have no time for childish rescinding—we remain priests of Jesus Christ forever.

I recall a prayer I used to say privately as a young seminarian during the years of my philosophical training. It is as clear to me today as it was yesterday. I was only nineteen or twenty. In the evening, after the long study hour and after the formal community night prayers, I would go privately to the front of the chapel very close to the tabernacle. And there before His tabernacle of imprisonment, in the darkness of the night and in the stillness of the quiet monastic surroundings, dressed in the black cassock, I would pray the prayer that the Lord had placed upon my heart: "O Lord, detach me from myself, that I may be attached only to You."

A man in the priesthood, in order to serve God and his people, must develop a Christ-centered character. If his character is erroneously centered elsewhere—perhaps in the pride and vanity of worldly endeavors, public acclaim, pursuit of knowledge for its own sake, and what have you—he will in the end have acquired only spiritual destitution and spiritual immaturity. These produce their own fruits: a character of emptiness and frustration, a personality rooted in envy, jealousy, condemnation, irrationality, and hatred. God, according to an old Spanish friend of mine, cannot live, cannot work, with such an indisposed vessel. It is always dark and lonely for one who lives away from Christ. A priest without a Christ-centered character is like the proverbial reed that is tossed hither and thither by every breeze. But if his character be centered in Christ, then such a one is like a sturdy oak. Regardless of age and circumstance, the sacred oil of holy anointing will remain always upon his soul.

Each priest is anointed with the Holy Spirit. Consider the words of Mary's *Magnificat*, as popularly rephrased: "The power of God has made me great, and my greatness stands alone above every other greatness." Is this not the song of gratitude that each priest must proclaim from his heart? On the day of his ordination, these thoughts overwhelm him. But to whom is this greatness due? Certainly not to any of us. It is due to a presence which is above us. It is the central idea of the Catholic priesthood. What the world honors in us is the Christ living in us, personifying Himself in time to the whole world, which He gave us as our parish.

The vital force that lives within me finds its roots in a personal love of the great High Priest Jesus Christ Himself, who made me His priest. God is a giver of gifts, and the greatest gift He could have granted mankind is the gift of His person in a chosen vessel. I therefore thank Him that from all eternity, notwithstanding the broken vessel of clay that is my humanity, He has chosen me. He, despite my frailty and fragility, has allowed me to be His visible instrument to walk among His people, to speak to them, to bless them, to teach, to preach, and to heal—to be in a very distinctive way His person, to act in His person, to continue in His person, to be His ambassador of truth and reconciliation. What an ineffable joy for a man destined in priesthood!

St. Paul tells us that to serve is to reign. Each priest serving God's community can say that he bears the world in his heart, and with Christ, and through Him, he can offer all to the Father. Nothing is more inspiring than the example of someone who truly burns out and is burned for the sake of the Lord. It is God's grace alone that allows the priest to encompass wholeheartedly and unreservedly the Master's Cross. It is God's grace alone that even musters him to embrace his death. It is His death, His Cross, His resurrection that offers to a broken humanity a ministry of healing, a ministry of intercession. Regardless of the cost, Paul's statement ultimately makes a lot of sense: "There is nothing I cannot master with the help of the One who gives me strength." (Ph. 4:13)

St. Gregory the Great ("Regula Pastoralis," I, I:PL, 77, 14.) says that the supreme art is the direction of souls. His statement indicates that the priestly power finds its expression through many diverse ways and whatever ways that are good and utilized by the priest enhance the special care of the salvation of others. It brings to them truth, love, and holiness, and this produces them as a people of God, building up the unity of the Church.

The priest is called to serve with his charism of priesthood. The priest is called to an apostolate. The priest's apostolic life flows from a soul of an apostolate, namely a life of inner prayer, to a world that is holistically broken and in salvific need. The miracle of miracles, the wonderment of wonderments of a priest's external ministry is impelled by his own inner experience of God, his own baptism of the spirit. So impelled, he must go forth to tell the world about his own wonderful voyage of discovery. In so doing, the priest of Jesus not only sends up to God the infinite tribute of adoration, thanksgiving, and reparation due Him, but he also, through his ministry of intercession, brings down a host of divine graces and precious blessings. Through his ordination powers, the priest personifies Christ, the merciful Jesus, who forgives sinners, purifies their souls, and directs them toward heaven. Through the administration of the sacrament of penance, like his Master, the Good Shepherd, who pursues as a Hound of Heaven the lost sheep, he brings them back to the fold and leads them to Christ's embrace. Through the priest, Christ's people are fed with the Eucharist of the Lord's body and blood, a sacrifice of victimhood of love.

One must never divest God's people of the healthy psychological processes that lead to the recognition of truth. People need external signs. The charisms serve as signs by which Christ is visibly experienced. The people of God are touched by Christ, as the priest who serves them personifies the compassionate Jesus, Who in His own lifetime blessed the inhabitants of Galilee, Samaria, Judea. When Jesus made sacred all things of the earth, He made visible the Father's presence. The Holy Spirit continues to nourish and sanctify the Father's human creation as he continues to make the Christ visible. The Christ living in the priest becomes a channel of the Holy Spirit. And so, like his Master, the priest helps the poor, consoles the afflicted, visits the sick and suffering, assists the dying to face the world of eternity. From the pulpit, his priestly heart and mind, having been first nourished at the feet of his living Christ, preach truth, life, a doctrine of true faith, hope, and love.

By his own example, he frees God's people from satanic influence unto a liberation of true ethical and moral behavior which conducts the human person to his true dignity: happiness, peace and salvation.

As the snows of many winters whiten the hair of the priest, as one's back becomes bent and as the young years of zeal and activity give way to the various stages of growing old, the priest prepares himself for the final day to face his beloved Christ. He is consumed by the life and interest of the Christ Who dwelled so vividly in him. At the final transition from earth to eternity, at the borderline crossing from here to eternity, the priest realizes that he as a man was consecrated.

There cascade through his mind a host of flashing scenes that were part of his life, incidents that were presented to him by God for his healing priestly blessing. He, in a flicker of a last human perception, realizes that he has passed through the world, a world that God permitted him to touch, a world in which he was to have done good, a world in which he was to seek no human reward except that reward which would become the crown and glory of his consecrated life. The human good that he performed will be remembered by a host of many: the poor, the suffering, the brokenhearted, the sick, the children whom he caressed. On the other hand, as is a mark of humanity, he may be forgotten. But he will not be forgotten by the Lord, Who welcomes him into the City of God: "Come to Me, good and faithful servant."

It is always an embarrassing situation for one to speak of oneself and one's inner thoughts. It is far more embarrassing to speak of the intimacies transpiring between God and the human soul, a precious union indeed. And so it is with myself. I find it somewhat difficult and most humbling to speak of the events and transpirings of my spiritual intimacies with God. Nevertheless, after speaking with my own bishop and Ordinary only a few months ago, I felt a personal need to convey to him that life, though apparently long in vision, is nevertheless very brief in its breath. As I had expressed to him, life for me, too, is rapidly passing. Its earthly end, with its eternal beginning, may also be close at hand for me. My soul belongs to God; my life belongs to the Church.

The Church breathes its spirit for every age. Every age, through God's grace shepherds its people through visible signs. One of the most precious concerns of God is the ministry to the sick, to the poor, and to the suffering. When God chooses a man or a woman to attend to such needs, there is a tremendous intimacy, an intimacy so secretive that even the soul so endowed with God's presence through a distinctive gift becomes astounded and perplexed. Yet each soul endowed must surpass all feelings and sentiments of personal embarrassment and present to the living Church on earth the soul of its apostolate.

Many have asked me to unfold the soul that guides my own behavior in relationship to the Apostolate of Prayer for Healing. And so in writing some of these experiences, I share them with the general public but in particular with those who share brotherhood with me in the sacred bond of Holy Orders. In my own words to my bishop: "That which God has done to me I must now share with the Church at large and with my brother priests, that they, too, may muster from within their own inner sanctum those natural gifts that God has given to them." May the thoughts I share in the chapters of this book enrich and encourage those who read them. May they surrender their natural qualities and gifts to the Almighty Giver of all gifts. In so doing, may each soul who is willing to step out in faith for the sake of Christ and for His cause, the Church, realize that their natural gifts are the foundation for charisms that personify the presence of Christ among His people.

And so I speak to you of an enslaving conviction of my own life, that there is a soul of the apostolate, an interior life of deep unity with God, that must precede every external apostolate. It is a life of prayer by which God is real with His presence, by which one lives constantly, night and day, morning and noon, seven days a week, every moment of life until the very end of earthly existence opens the portals for the beginning of eternal life. Every man's spirituality is the soul of his behavior, and that is God alone. In translation, this signifies not action, not contemplation, not works, not rest, not this or that particular thing, but God alone in everything, God in anything, God in His will, God in other men, God present in one's own soul. This has deeper implications, that when God alone reigns supreme in a soul it is no longer the human being that lives, but it is the spirit of God urging one to do God's will and even to suffer whatever God wills.

At the concluding session of one of my last crusades at Manhattan College, in New York, Auxiliary Bishop Francisco Garmendia stood before an assembly of eight thousand people. During the two previous days, before sixteen thousand people, he had witnessed the power of Jesus Christ alive in His Church. He witnessed the soul of the apostolate alive in me. He witnessed along with another auxiliary bishop of New York, Bishop Joseph Pernicone, the soul of the apostolate re-enkindling and recharging the souls of priests, sisters, brothers, and lay people. External manifestations were abundant. There was great spiritual renewal. The message of God the Father was alive in our modern day: "Yes, God loved the world so much that He gave His only Son, so that every one who believes in Him may not be lost but may have eternal life." (Jn. 3:16) In a tender but forceful voice, this simple and unpretentious but powerful Church prelate looked directly into my eyes as I sat there humbly among my brother priests after having ministered for three days to the brokenness of New York City. His voice, thundering forth like a voice from on high, proclaimed to the public and to me: "Ralph, my brother priest, you are simple and filled with faith. You truly have been called by God, not because of yourself but because God has called you to Himself to evangelize His people. Your ministry to the church of God is a pure ministry of evangelization. May God bless you and strengthen you to renew His Church. May you always be faithful to God and to the Church that you serve."

What Jesus has done to me is particular, is real: the ministry of evangelization and holistic healing. What Jesus has done to me is nothing else but what He had always planned for me to be. What Jesus has done to me He also wants to do and can do to each one of you who are reading my words, laity and clergy alike. To each one of you He can impart His Holy Spirit in a very different and in a very distinctive way proper to the very being that He created in each one of you. His grace will work upon your nature: It will embellish you, it will raise you up to the status of a charism. And that charism will be used for the building up of the broken body, the Church. This, in essence, is the measure of a spiritual vocation. The Second Letter from Paul to Timothy says: "This is why I am reminding you now to fan into a flame the gift that God gave you when I laid my hands on you." (2 Tm. 1:6)

Among the greatest gifts that God shares with man is the gift of friendship. This chapter, on priesthood, is very precious to me. Priests have ministered to me for fifty-two years of my life, and now I find it a joy and a privilege to be able to share in some way my ministry to priests in return. And so I have addressed this chapter and these thoughts not only to the laity—who by reading them may have a better conception of priesthood—but to all my brother priests, here and afar, young and old.

Many of you look upon me as someone special, someone different. Only by Christ's choosing has He allowed Himself to be "special" and "different" through me. Without this Christ I am an ordinary human being. But because of the Christ that has overpowered my life, I am a priest and I must live not for myself but to lead men to Christ. The priesthood which you and I share is a living sacrament. The priest is a man, a man whose father and mother we may know, yet through his ordination he becomes a sacrament of Christ. He has assumed a new character. He has been marked by a sign. That sign is the divine anointing of the Holy Spirit. "The Spirit of the Lord has been given to me, for he has anointed me." (Lk. 4:18) From that moment, he is Christ living among us. When the people give the priest the beautiful name of "Father" it is because they know that he has left everything in order to beget a higher life in them. "It is to the priest," says St. John Chrysostom, "that the spiritual procreation of souls was entrusted." Our parents beget us through the first life, the priest through the second.

If it is true that one thing only is necessary in life—the salvation of one's soul—then the priest is the most necessary one, because salvation is only through the priest. Christ, after His resurrection, did not confine His priesthood to a celestial intercession on our behalf. He has willed to exercise His priesthood here, in the world, through the priest.

Like you, Our Blessed Lord rested His eyes on me also. In the days of my boyhood He called me. Like you, I heard His voice, either directly in the depth of my heart through the inspiration of His divine grace, or through the medium of a good priest, a teacher, a friend. Like you, there were other boys around me who seemed to be more worthy than I was of the vocation to the holy priesthood, and better fitted for the fulfillment of its duties. Yet, unlike you and me, they were not called. From among countless souls, you and I had been set apart in God's eternal designs for the sacred and sublime office of the priesthood. We became objects of special care and love from our Divine Redeemer. We had not chosen Him, for we had no claim to so great a favor. He had chosen us out of His infinite kindness and mercy. "You did not choose me, no, I chose you; and I commissioned you to go out and bear fruit, fruit that will last." (Jn. 15:16)

> Boyhood dreams of long ago
> Saw an altar fair,
> Consecrated, trembling hands
> Lifted there in prayer.
> And those dreams have led me on,
> Dreamlike though they seemed,
> Now dear friend, thank God with me,
> I am what I dreamed.
> Other dreams have I today,
> Bright in spite of fears,
> That this human heart may be
> Christlike through the years.
> Think of me when on your knees
> That this dream come true,
> Bowed before that altar fair,
> There I'll think of you.

However vague and distant that first call may have been, it resounded in our souls. The invisible attraction of Christ's initial call became visible through His various influential attractions. They drew us nearer to the altar. We came into closer contact with the idea of the holy priesthood. As we yielded our nothingness to Him, He with His everything surrendered Himself to us, making out of our nothingness a new creation—an *alter Christus*. "*Vocavit me vocatione sua sancta*"—He called us into a holy vocation.

A priest is many things. In the eyes of early boyhood, he is someone who stands at the altar dressed in bright-colored vestments and speaks from the pulpit to a respectfully silent and hopefully attentive audience. He sits for hours in the confessional, hearing the sins of penitents and giving absolution. He baptizes the newly born and performs the ceremony of marriage. He is sent for when someone is dangerously ill. He reads mass for the sick and the suffering and the dead. He is clearly someone who is invested with special power and authority. He definitely exerts a great influence on his community.

Such is the priest as he appears in the public exercise of his sacred function. Some never go beyond this external and superficial knowledge of a priest. It is possible, however, to form a much more exalted and complete idea of what a priest is.

As individuals, with all our human frailty, but made divine by God's anointing, we priests aim to conquer the world for Christ. We go forth to change the world, hoping not to be changed by it. The never-ending battle rages. Satan and his forces attack endlessly; but Christ is continually the Victor. With love for Christ in our hearts, with zeal tempered by prudence, with knowledge equipping our minds, with character in our will, we are thrust into the arena of man's chaotic world.

What can we priests call on for daily strength, for survival? Christ, our life, said: "Watch and pray." That is the answer. That is the means for us to persevere in our noble vocation. Christ is constantly in union with the presence of His Father. His life was a personification of prayer. He is a Priest. He is the High Priest.

Who can conceive of a priest who is not holy, not prayerful? The priest is uniquely a man of prayer both public and private.

In his liturgical prayer life—the Mass, Divine Office, and administration of the sacraments—the priest is the official minister of his bride, of his Church. He is the intermediary, like his Master, between his people and his God. In his private devotions, meditations, and spiritual reading, in his daily Holy Hour, he seeks to perfect his own soul, to provide new strength for his work for others. "No one gives what he does not possess." (*Nemo dat quod non habet*—Latin adage)

When God gives a vocation, God does not leave that vocation unsustained. God sustains us each day through actual graces for each moment of that day. By these daily graces, a priest—who inevitably must be attacked both by his own humanity and from the stress and pressures of a modern world—will be able to renew his sacred commitment. His private prayer, his meditative consideration of the exalted dignity of the priesthood, is the soul of his apostolate. These reflections should constantly speak to him. They should continue to energize his public and official prayer presentation. There is no other way that a priest can remain faithful to the Lord. There is no other way that he can refresh himself with the ideal and aims that marked his early days of youthful vigor. All other means, regardless of how good they may be, such as the use of modern psychological techniques, are only secondary. A priest who daily kneels before the tabernacle of Christ, who preaches the unchanged message of the Cross and the Blood, as great men of all ages—Augustine, St. John of the Cross, Archbishop Fulton J. Sheen, Billy Graham—will always know who they are, what they are for, and Who their God is. The single element necessary for the priest to be like Christ among the people is authentic non-neurotic holiness, the simplicity of being, *nothing else.*

If the priest does not personify his Master by his behavior or words, he has betrayed his mission, and therefore his vocation. His ministry, a mere peripheral expression, becomes a church built upon sand. His priesthood is of little use either to himself (in fact, a burden) or to the people. His people, observing and hearing him, will taunt him, not without reason. They will object: "They claim to have knowledge of God but the things they do are nothing but a denial of him." (Tt. 1:16) The people will reject his teaching and fail to profit by his life as a priest. If holiness is neglected, if it is absent, then the priest cannot be in any way the salt of the earth, for what is itself contaminated is quite unfitted for preserving soundness. When sanctity is lacking, corruption is soon present.

Jesus said: "It is good for nothing, and can only be thrown out to be trampled underfoot by men." (Mt. 5:13)

What essentially is this necessary holiness? It is simply character, based on belief, conviction, determination, decisiveness, each second, each breath of our lives until the very end. Holiness of life is the result of character. It is the *fruit of our will*. God Himself supplies us with a tremendous provision, so that we may never, unless we so will it, be without grace. And if, in momentary weakness, we become like Peter in his denial, in his fall, then like Peter in his return we will perceive the endless penetrating glance of the love of a wounded Jesus saying: "Come, I still love you. Arise, take my hand. I am He Whom you seek." And with that Peter, whom all of us are so naturally drawn to with awe, love, respect, and consolation, we hear said to us: ". . . your new birth was not from any mortal seed but from the everlasting word of the living and eternal God. All flesh is grass and its glory like the wild flower's. The grass withers, the flower falls, but the word of the Lord remains for ever." (1 P. 1:23–25)

The Church will never alter her requisite for priests of mission and ministry. She holds in constant esteem the profound and supernatural mission which the Lord gave to us and which St. Paul so clearly states: "People must think of us as Christ's servants, stewards entrusted with the mysteries of God." (1 Co. 4:1) This is what Christians and non-Christians look for when they seek the sincerity of Christ's presence. This is what people demand of us who walk in the person of Christ. They have a right to make this demand. It is what each priest and minister, each servant of the Most High, must fulfill if he is to be truly conscious of his own dignity and responsibility to lead all forms of human society back to God.

Many people who see us as priests following the obedient and celibate Nazarene appear to regard us with a kind of sadness, to see us, as Paul says, as "fools for Christ." But are we really fools? Some say we have to be a bit different, perhaps even odd, to be priests. But I don't believe that is true. I've known many outstanding priests and bishops. Some were ex-big-league ballplayers; some were artists and musicians. Some, like Father Willy Doyle, S.J., were chaplains in the armed forces. Others, like Father George Keerr, formerly captain of the Boston College team that beat Tennessee in the Sugar

Bowl, were definitely all-American guys. And from the ranks of untold Irish families, many a policeman has left his civic rank to join the ranks of Christ. Countless ex-servicemen are now fighting as soldiers of Christ. As young men they fought in Iwo Jima, Guadalcanal, New Guinea. Many who risked their lives on the beaches of Cassino and Normandy now are priests.

Father John O'Neill, from Providence, Rhode Island, once commented, "Some people figure a priest is a fellow who never did like girls and probably hates babies." But the reality is that a priest is not a priest at all if he hates anybody. Our Lord Jesus Christ loved women. He saved an adulterous girl from the Pharisees. He gave her hope for a better tomorrow. To the woman at the well He gave the source of living waters: faith. And to that broken flower, Magdalene, He changed not the natural emotion of love, which she had abused, but the object of her emotion. He gave her Himself, and from that moment on He was her way, her truth, her all. As for children, how can you be a priest if you dislike them? Christ said: "Let the little ones come to me."

During the past seven years, in answer to the profound needs of our age, God has made Himself known as the Healer of Mankind in a much more vivid way. He has been using me as a channel of transmission of this grace. Through the healing ministry, the Lord has also used me to speak and deliver His Father's message. He has permitted me to serve with a strength beyond my own, a strength wholly provided by God. To be specially called by God and to fulfill that call adequately, the one chosen must yield and surrender to the divine will. Without obedience, a priest is totally ineffective.

The yielding and the surrender encompass one's whole life, from the crib to the tomb. When I ask myself how this all began I see that when I was young many possibilities were present. Each one was good. One path could have led to a marriage and family, to a career in medicine or art. The talents and the qualifications were there. Adults who took an interest in me attempted to steer me along that path. The other path, which was presented to me somberly, and was perhaps less exciting and promising, had a mysterious impact on the inner sanctum of my soul. Its value, its promise lay in the unending truth. God did not seem a sad God, after all.

As I looked along those paths in order to discern the true way, I realized that, whichever one I chose, I would have to give up something, and either way I saw rewards. But down deep in my young boy's heart, there paraded before my mind such figures as Father Flanagan, of Boys Town. He stood before me as a giant of a priest: warm, compassionate, intimate with God, caring, willing to take risks. And often I recalled the many words and the behavior of visiting missionary priests. I called those priests God's troubadours. How forcefully they spoke of God needing men who would willingly sacrifice everything to give men, women, and children a new baptism of God's life.

Words express thoughts, and this leads to actions. The words of the missionary priest seemed to challenge me—a challenge for Christ. I liked that. And so the thought became action. The voice of God called me and led me to the Roman Catholic priesthood. Man may not touch that which God has willed. Off I went to the seminary with determination in my mind and love within my heart.

The seminary was tough going. But then, what isn't if it be truly worthwhile? I saw a lot of fellow seminarians arrive and leave. Some cracked under the strict regimen. Some of our relatives and friends told us that we were crazy to lock ourselves up inside a seminary to become priests. But God kept us going. After a while, the worldly sights and the worldly sounds that had once intrigued us grew flat and empty. Prayer and knowledge became our constant companions. Our minds were enriched by the study of languages, philosophy, psychology, literature, theology. Our prayer life of walking intimately with God reflected the purpose of our calling.

I loved all these experiences. I wanted holiness above everything else. Knowledge and science would be necessary to a certain degree but holiness was the key. A priest who combines holiness with knowledge becomes Christ among his people. I am inspired by the thoughts of John Paul II: "A priest is a man of prayer, a man of knowledge. A priest from his prayer and knowledge bears strong convictions of faith, strong stands on morality. A priest is seen by the human family as friend, humble pastor, leader, man of vision, man of compassion, man of understanding, a priestly man having time for his people. A priest schooled in suffering and adversity becomes the defender and promoter of the beauty of Christian faith and tradition because he is a man who is strong spiritually, a man keen and profound in pastoring, a person of great heart, a person of great goodness. A priest then can go forth into the arena of humanity as a supporter of human rights, as a spokesman for religious minorities. The Church then can gladly proclaim that it has ordained men who are empowered with trust and courage. It has ordained each priest to be ready to suffer for Christ and His Church, even imprisonment and the shedding of blood. A priest should bless the world." Such a priest truly can proclaim the significant words of Ruth to Naomi:

"Wherever you go, I will go,
wherever you live, I will live.
Your people shall be my people,
and your God, my God." (Rt. 1:16)

Pray for us. . . .

Lord Jesus Christ, Good Shepherd, you laid down your life for your sheep. We commend our priests to your loving care. Humbly they walk in your sacred footsteps, devoted to the Church and the service of God's people. You are their hope in time of discouragement. You are strength in their human weakness. As they minister to us, Lord, help us to reach out to them.

Remove their doubts, as you did those of Thomas. Deepen their faith and forgive their sins as you forgave repentant Peter. And as you gave John, the beloved disciple, to your mother at the foot of the cross—so also entrust your priests to the tender embrace of Mary, Mother of the Church and Queen of the Clergy.   Amen

(Prayer for priests
by Bishop Joseph F. Maguire,
Bishop of Springfield, Mass.)

8

WHY THIS MAN, O LORD?

"Ecce ego, Domine: quia vocasti me."
"Here I am, since you called me." (1 S. 3:6)

We are called, we are chosen, we are life to one another. "Yes, God loved the world so much that he gave his only Son, so that every one who believes in him may not be lost but may have eternal life. For God sent his Son into the world not to condemn the world, but so that through him the world might be saved." (Jn. 3:16–17)

To answer the question "Why this man, O Lord?" one with spiritual vision must penetrate the words of St. John. His statement is impregnated with the concept that the Father loves the world. Through His loving the world, His loving us, both you and I are drawn into a personal relationship with God, ourselves, and the world. Furthermore, in so loving the world, the Father calls you and me to experience Him. And in so doing, the Father convinces you and me of His love as He sends His Son among us. The Father's love for us, His call to us, cannot involve the stagnancy of a status quo. The Father who intends to renew the face of the earth through His Son, Jesus Christ, intends to promulgate by proper propaganda. And so, therefore, the Father not only loves, not only calls, but He also shares you and me with others by our witness. He calls us to be a star of vision, a voice of evangelization. Whom are we to witness? We are to witness God yesterday, today, and always. We are to witness His faithfulness, His concern, and His person. To whom are we to witness? We are to witness to God's children, all of mankind, regardless of nationality and creed. What are we to witness? We are to witness the spirituality of the second Pentecost.

Throughout time and space, God has never ceased to associate men and women with His Son in the redemption of the world. This work of redemption is still in progress. The search for unity, truth, charity, justice and peace goes on and on until time be no more.

Now, more than ever, Christ finds Himself asking His disciples: "Why have you been standing here idle all the day?" The Church is stunned by man's refusal to help. It is perhaps time for our human family to ask: "What does Christ want from us specifically? What does Christ want from me, who have received so much from an abundant Father, a saving Christ, and a sanctifying Spirit?" The answer is that the Trinity wants us unto Themselves.

Christ as Teacher, Preacher, and Healer, Christ as Saviour and Redeemer, extends Himself through gifts. In a special way, He transmits Himself into the heart of His renewal. He imbues it with the person of Himself and of the Father and the Holy Spirit. It is this Holy Spirit Who anoints generous souls in response to God's call, whether to the religious life or to some other life. He calls all to serve: sinners and saints. He calls mankind to nurse mankind with the balm of heaven's healing love.

Truly, to serve is to reign. Give your hands to help others; give your heart to love them. Our life of service is as necessary as the work itself. In heaven we shall see how much we owe to those whom we have served: for they have helped us serve the Christ better. We find Christ in the poor, the suffering, the sick, the sinner, the saint; in the black man, the white man, the Oriental; in the Catholic, the Protestant, the Jew, and the pagan.

When Our Blessed Lord first called Peter and the other apostles to Himself, He said that from now on they would catch souls instead of fish. The responsibility increased: That is, they themselves, with the heart and mind of Christ burning within them, would multiply Christ's fold.

The Christian law teaches that the higher we are called, the lower we are to become, and this is the beauty and encouragement of human frailty, of human brokenness. All of us have the opportunity to make ourselves be what God wants us to be. We must never forget that we are vessels of clay in the Potter's hand, and if there should ever be a moment when we are dejected by our human weaknesses, let us remember Jeremiah: "And whenever the vessel he was making came out wrong, as happens with the clay handled by potters, he would start afresh and work it into another vessel, as potters do." (Jr. 18:4–5)

Regardless of the height of our callings, of our specific charisms, the euphoria initially experienced will eventually be recognized as responsibility. God will keep the weight of responsibility before us ever constantly. His tool, His chisel is the virtue of humility. And so, in a very short time, we must come down from the mountain of transfiguration. In a very short time a disciple, an apostle, a follower of Christ discovers that he is no different from before, that the clay is just as weak as ever and that the esteem people give to him or her is not necessarily the way the Lord looks upon this responsibility. Y E T , G O D C A L L S . And we must respond. "O Lord, I, Your servant, hear Your cry, I hear Your voice. I will answer Your cry. I will communicate with Your voice. I will accept Your call, the call that ever beckons me on as a Hound of Heaven."

The worth of a follower of Christ is measured by his donation to life, not merely its duration. God will judge us not on what we appear to accomplish in our given time, but on *how much* we reflected Him, not only in a work, but in word and life. He will ask us if we spoke His message through our hearts and voice; He will seek the visible sign of His image manifested to a people craving for external signs. When the hourglass of life ceases, we will be judged not by how long we served, nor on how much we did, but on whether or not people saw and felt Christ among us.

And so in answering the question "Why this man, O Lord?" I have shared with you the mind of God as He creates, loves, renews, and requests. When a gift is authentic and true, the person who is gifted responds with a spontaneity that is beyond one's normal human powers—a response directed and produced by the Trinity, through the sanctifying agency of the Holy Spirit.

With reference to the special gifts of healing with which God has endowed me, the only obligation I have toward God and toward a broken humanity is to step out in faith upon the waters for the miracle that comes from the Christ. I have absolutely no power and strength of my own; but simply through my own broken and weak humanity, a more vivifying power, a supernatural entity anoints and overpowers me to accomplish the work of the Lord. For this, God granted me life; for this, God called; for this, God trained and embellished; for this was I ordained a priest of Jesus Christ.

There are times when I do wonder why the gift was granted to me. As I look back on friends and acquaintances, I see that there were so many others who were probably more efficient and capable. During rare free moments I amuse myself by seeking an appropriate answer. When they come from God, the answers are, I assure you, most humble. The finest answer I draw forth is that in my own weakness and brokenness, I, too, needed the Wounded Healer's love, and in my availability to be doctored by the Divine Physician, His own healing love renewed me to witness the healing bond to my fellow men.

And yet, perhaps it was because I always wanted to be available to the Lord. Further, perhaps it was because I really believed in Christ —that He lives, that He is truly the Son of God, born of the Virgin Mary, who suffered and died under a time-serving politician called Pilate, arose from the dead, and lives in His Church.

And then, perhaps, as I am so often told, I may have been more naïve to believe that He is not a sad God, after all. Yet once in His lifetime Jesus saved a wedding party from its sadness by changing water into wine. And because of that, everyone was happy—including the uninvited apostles.

Again, perhaps I was simple enough to believe that this marvelous Galilean did say to the dead Lazarus: "Lazarus, here! Come out!" (Jn. 11:43) and that restoration to life was a true fact. Above all, that which touched my heart most about this intriguing heavenly visitor to earth was that He loved children, cured the blind, and made the lame walk and run again.

Or, because of my philosophical background, I may have been demanding God to respect His own creation of psychological processes to truth. That God, Who was invisible, could become visible through signs and wonders. And so the answer, in the final analysis, really is founded upon humility: *"Domine, non sum dignus*—Lord, I am not worthy. But, Lord, if you can take this nothingness, then make me into a new creation for Your glory and for the welfare of Your Church."

True humility must be forged and tried by the fires of discernment and authority. That forging and trial must be tempered by the utmost respect for Christ's earthly representatives, the superiors of the Church. Being just a small priest without the fullness of consecrated priesthood and being ordained by him who has the fullness of the episcopacy, I thereupon become only the extension of his responsibility as shepherd. He who bears the fullness of the Spirit, as invested in him through authority, needs continued charisms in the members he has ordained to perpetuate the presence of Christ among the people.

The rock of the Church is built upon obedience, and not upon visible manifestations of charisms. The visible signs however, flow forth smoothly, positively, and appropriately when legitimate authority sends them forth with the voice of Christ: "Go out to the whole world; proclaim the Good News to all creation. He who believes and is baptized will be saved; he who does not believe will be condemned. These are the signs that will be associated with believers: in my name they will cast out devils; they will have the gift of tongues; they will pick up snakes in their hands, and be unharmed should they drink deadly poison; they will lay their hands on the sick, who will recover." (Mk. 16:15–18)

Christ Himself was obedient unto the death of the cross. When one loses his life for God, he will gain it. In reality what is taking place through my particular call and personal response is that God has raised up another medium for His communicative life to flow to His people.

With such an extraordinary gift of healing that God has granted to me, a far greater gift was given to me in the person of my Ordinary and local superior, Bishop Bernard J. Flanagan. As it was hard for me to understand what God had suddenly done to my life in 1976, so, too, it caused perplexity among those who had to oversee both me personally and the welfare and protection of the Church. Was this gift authentic? Was the gift authentic in the priest? The priest himself was authentically ordained. Were the gifts of healing from the Lord? The priest in question was ordained validly in the Lord. Was the loyalty of the Church's charisms being upheld for the community's good by this priest? The priest himself was conscious of his own nothingness, and his intentions and behavior were always loyal to the Church. He was enriched in the service of its people. Was God choosing a cornerstone—simple, yet solid? Would this cornerstone be another rock for the building up of the Church?

The priest in question had been no stranger to pain and sorrow, to prayer, patience, and perseverance. He himself had often been ground into human dust and quarried from the Rock of Ages. With moral certitude, and strengthened by years of guidance, this simple priest was ready to be used by the hand of the Church. And such was discerned and approved by a shepherd of Jesus Christ, Bishop Flanagan. Through his own moments of perplexity, but with the consolation of long hours of prayer, observation, and prudence, Bishop Flanagan saw God's hand raised to bless both his local church of Worcester, Massachusetts, and an outreach propagation of the faith in a ministry of which the Church was in need. So began the Office of the Apostolate of Prayer for Healing.

A priest never touches reality until he touches a soul. We are not the agents who save souls. We do not cause results. Actually, all we are at best are instruments of God's love among men. Souls are our interest—their salvation as persons, whole persons, must be uppermost in our minds, and this includes their healing of spirit, soul, and body. Jesus did this because He came not to save souls; He came to save *persons*.

Although the gift may be beautiful for the people because it gives them renewed hope, faith, and love, nevertheless it weighs heavily upon me; my body, my spirit, my soul, and my heart. There is no doubt that I am convinced that I am only one human being, subject to time, circumstance, space, human fatigue, and human frailties. I cannot reach everyone. The cries and tears of so many people cause me to realize evermore than before that by God's permission the world has become my parish. I bear the world in my heart, and with Christ and through Him I offer all to the Father. I do feel people's pain. There permeates throughout my being a tremendous desire to absorb the warmth of their tears flowing upon my shoulders. I want to touch their hands; I want to be one with their pain; I seek to embrace their broken humanity and through my own broken humanity, blessed by grace, to touch theirs with His divinity.

Is it not true that sometimes we priests, because of our background, culture, and training, are afraid to touch another human being? We are afraid to put our arms around a troubled person, man or woman, afraid to express divinity through humanity? Yet this is what Jesus did.

I remember walking one day toward the confessional box of a

church. I had never been there previously. I noticed an impressive painting hanging upon an adjacent wall. With my artist's eyes I appreciated the artistic genius of the painter, who transmitted the impressive image of the compassionate Jesus embracing a teenager. Jesus hugged him tight. He received his tears. He extended His healing grace. And a wandering, adventurous teenager, one lost in the quagmire of sin and the obscurity of a darkened forest, suddenly was renewed for the new chapters of an unfolding autobiography. Blushing a bit, I smiled and walked to the communion rail before the tabernacle. I dared to speak to the Master, but all that I could say was "Thank you, Jesus. Thank you for letting me be human."

How often God attempts to continually sensitize us by His presence dwelling in others. Jesus was truly human; Christ Jesus was truly divine. As I was about to arise from my knees, I thought I heard a voice say: "Stay on, stay on, for I have a message for you. I want you to feel my people's loneliness; I want you to experience their brokenness. I do not want you only to proclaim healings, to preach, and to teach. I want you to be one with my people. I want you to be sensitized in every aspect to their pain. I want you to show them that the sadness and tears of their lives are heard by my Father and that with perseverance, prayer, patience, and penance, I will wipe away their tears."

As I admitted earlier, I cannot bear to see other persons in pain, especially children. I somehow feel at one with their pain. I experience their pain as if it were mine. The Lord used the pain He permitted me to experience for the purpose of sensitizing me to the world of pain and anguish—to the dregs and brokenness of humanity. All things considered, God was preparing the soil for the apostolate.

We priests belong to the people; we are theirs, and they have a right to us. Moreover, our vocational response is "*Victima— sacerdos*" (priest). In our priesthood, what else are we supposed to do but to be a priest, all priest, twenty-four hours a day, every day of our life until we breathe with Christ His last word: "*Pater, in manus tuas commendo spiritum meum. . . . Consummatum est*—Father, into Your hands I commend my spirit. . . . [It is consummated.]" (Lk. 23:46 NAB)

My schedule, too, is overwhelming. Time is not my own. The apostolate to the sick requires my constant dedication, both in my home diocese of Worcester and in other dioceses, through the increasingly overwhelming requests of bishops. In humility, they desire to feed their people with the same Christ of yesterday, today, and forever.

The needs and the cries of the people keep me constantly alert to both prayer and external ministry. For one so meticulous and neat as myself, I am often amused at how God has broken me of these traits. Traveling to and fro, I see that ordinary, common difficulties are made easy, and that one can learn to live with little and with what is essential. Living out of a suitcase most of the time is like the experience of an itinerant missionary. Nevertheless, it is done out of love for a cause. Better still, I do it unselfishly for the love of God and because it grants me the opportunity to be an extension of Him to His people, not only here in Worcester but wherever invitation and authority welcome us. That's a great reward!

But all these external demands must have a soul. The soul of the external apostolate, for both myself and my staff, rests in the heart of prayer, where heart speaks to heart, God and man. Whatever free time I can find, besides the stringently imposed daily standard hours of ascetical discipline, I spend in prayer, almost always in front of the tabernacle. It is there that most inspirations come from the Lord. Before His feet and from His Sacred Heart, I receive physical, spiritual, and mental strength in order to carry on the mission of Christ.

Those are splendid moments at night before the Lord—in the darkness of a chapel, in the quiet of a church, in the requiem of silent prayer. A priest, a nun, a layman, a friend, or even a stranger can become acquainted with this wandering Divine Troubadour, this King who always has time for an audience. When one kneels before the tabernacle, especially in the hours of the night, only the flickering of a candle burns away. It seems to tell the visitor that God has not forgotten him.

When carrying the pain and anguish of the apostolate that accompanies the gift that God has blessed me with, I am sustained by the example of Simon of Cyrene, who aided Our Lord with the cross. At first ignorant of the gift of cross bearing, he recoiled from its burden. Being forced because he was available, he looked into the Master's eyes. Within that moment of gaze, his burden became God's invitation to share the burden, the bearing of a broken world. At times I feel at one with the African Simon of Cyrene, but I hear the Master asking me: "Ralph, will you help me unselfishly, unreservedly? Will you help me to sanctify that portion of humanity that I desire to be redeemed in your lifetime? Will you allow me to use you to bring brothers and sisters together into unity?"

To such a pleading Sacred Heart I could not but say: Yes. Who would not be so moved by His gaze? The eyes of the crucified Jesus have always spoken to me more fluently than His voice: "You are Mine. You are Mine." Yes, like every chosen soul, like every priest, like every religious man and woman, I became His, I hope not only in time but forever in the agelessness of eternity. He gave Himself to me. Should I not then respond with the giving of myself? If we refuse, He will hound us as the "Hound of Heaven." But in the ultimate end the chase and the capture will be completely His.

One of those moments of utmost preciousness to me is that which every priest considers to be the best part of his day. It is what every priest is ordained for; to kneel and to stand, to pray with Christ as an *alter Christus* at the altar of sacrifice. This is daily Mass. I cannot conceive of a priest without his daily celebration of Mass, as I cannot conceive of a priest who does not pray. For me and for every priest, for those in city life, in country parishes, in jungles and forests, in concentration camps, behind the Iron Curtain, in Australia, Europe, the Americas, Asia, and Africa, the Holy Sacrifice of the Mass is our life. It is the very essence of priesthood, because true religion is founded at the altar. Everything else—teaching, preaching, and charism—are only by-products stemming out as expressions of divine actual grace transmitted through the Eucharistic Sacrifice. The priest, in the Sacrifice of the Eucharist, is doing that which Christ did best when He offered Himself to the Father for the redemption of man. Man has a Divine Intecessor. Man is forgiven; man is healed. During those sacred moments of daily Mass, an utmost reverence enslaves me, as it does all priests who realize that they are touching the Lord.

Life for us is at the foot of the altar, before the Eucharistic presence. Here our pain, frustration and doubts—through humility— speak eloquently to the Master in His tabernacle of love. They speak to Him of our brokenness, of our desire to serve, of our will to please Him, of our dreams, our fears, our searchings; yes, even of our logic, our reasoning, be it clear or perplexed, of our inner conflicts, our solace, our discoveries, and our answers.

Before the Lord each day we sentinels of the Lord enjoy precious moments of yet another experience of love. This is the daily Holy Hour. Within those precious moments the heart of man speaks to the heart of God—first by speaking to the Master and then, like Nicodemus, by listening. Precisely therein lies the core, the soul, of the priest. These intimate rendezvous are extremely precious, and the one enjoying them almost feels a personal jealousy toward any form of human intrusion. The experience of the Holy Hour could be likened to a private audience in a selected and far-off holy ground. It is like an enclosed garden wherein the human heart, much as wintered soil hardened and crusted by the harshness of past months, is tilled, seeded, watered and touched anew by the divine heart, right at its core.

In further answering the question "Why this man, O Lord?" another part of the holistic surrender to God must be considered. Many inquire as to how the gift operates through me. My answer is drawn from theology and philosophy, coupled intimately under what theology calls *gratia supplet naturam*—grace working, embellishing nature. This truly is a charism. Natural virtues and qualities are the basis upon which God transcends the ordinary into the extraordinary, the natural into the supernatural. It is grace working upon a grace by Him who is the Giver of all graces. In order to serve the Lord, one must be ready to surrender his gifts.

Christian virtue surpasses purely natural qualities in the very identical manner and proportion that divine grace surpasses human nature, both in power and in excellence. When divine grace works and acts in us, it neither destroys nor supplants man's nature. In actuality, what it does is correct and guide natural powers, natural inclinations. It assists and raises and perfects our natural gifts.

Our cooperation with God, with His grace, is nothing more than submitting ourselves as prepared soil. God's grace waters this well-prepared soil and fructifies it, and the more abundant becomes the spiritual harvest which the soil produces.

No one should ever think that by applying oneself assiduously to the practice of Christian virtues and to the fulfillment of religious duties, he or she should neglect the cultivation of the purely natural gifts which he or she has received from the Author of life. We are not allowed to become stagnant, apathetic; we are not allowed to leave unproductive and futile our powers or our respective beings.

Our bodies, our minds, our hearts were gifts in the natural order, from God. He has entrusted them to us. Our response is one of moral obligation to direct and develop these to such a point as to make them serve God, to give Him praise and glory.

In turn, our own spiritual progress and the good of our fellow men ensues. God made this emphatically clear through His Son, Jesus, when Our Blessed Lord spoke in the parable of the talents. (Mt. 25:14–30) In so doing we beautify and raise our human, fallen nature. We restore it to its original beauty and state of perfection as it came forth from the Creator's hands.

And finally, as we answer the question "Why this man, O Lord?" above all else, one who is called by God realizes that all glory and honor is to be given to the Trinity: that God the Father is Lord of all creation; that Jesus Christ is Lord of all redemption; that the Holy Spirit is Lord and agent of the Father and the Son in sanctification, and this is the foundation of the ministry of service.

Throughout the active ministry I repeatedly emphasize that God must be given the glory and the credit. Without faith in God the Father, who made Himself visible through His Son, Jesus Christ, and who continues His presence through the Holy Spirit, all the events and manifestations of my ministry would be a message without meaning, a heart without love, a body without a soul.

I am deeply grateful to God that during the past twenty-five years of my priesthood, he has used me to influence, motivate, and redirect countless souls to a renewal of spiritual, psychological, and bodily health. A dominant theme in my ministry: A man void of God is the profoundest of life's tragedies. I wanted to be used by Him to fill that void.

During the past seven years I have seen many experience personal surrender and positive commitment to God. Human brokenness has yielded up its emptiness to become filled by the divine plan. As each one of us becomes the best we can become through the use of our "natural" gifts, each one of us is touched to the point of surrendering to the Divine. Through human agents, the invisible becomes visible (*invisibilia per visibilia*). Man renders himself able to recognize God's concern and love for each human being in each circumstance. What a powerful responsibility this message is!

God alone "chooses and selects those whom He wills, and according to His own measure." God alone prepared, directed, and unfolded, through time and circumstances, the seemingly ordinary events that combined to make me into His distinctive tool—a tool fashioned to serve mankind's contemporary need for healing and restoration. Through this human instrument, God—Who is the Gift—continues to make His divine presence alive and relevant to all peoples. Wounded seekers discover the Divine Wounded Healer. The Divine Wounded Healer conveys Himself as the God who became man that man might become God. "Yes, God loved the world so much that he gave his only Son, so that everyone who believes in him may not be lost but may have eternal life." (Jn. 3:16)

This book, therefore, is before anything else a *deliberate attempt to give an exposition of God's love for man*. It aims to show how God, through a gift of healing, flows forth His love and mercy to the broken body of the Church, *to every man, woman, and child*, regardless of race and creed, regardless of individual denomination. It is God the Father renewing His children: ". . . while they, going out, preached everywhere, the Lord working with them and confirming the word by the signs that accompanied it." (Mk. 16:20)

This book is also an illumination of a Christian and Catholic priest's spirituality. Particularly, it arises from God's universal invitation to each soul to perfect itself as adequately as possible: "Be you holy as your heavenly Father is holy." It expounds God's constant attempt to empty me, His priest, of myself through trial and circumstance, so as to dispose me to be a better servant, a more receptive vessel for His fullest indwelling. God's dynamics always utilize the virtue of humility to reduce one into a nonentity, so to speak, so that the one chosen for a prominent distinctive mission becomes an authentic ambassador: ". . . and he has entrusted to us the news that they are reconciled. So we are ambassadors for Christ; it is as though God were appealing through us. . . ." (2 Co. 5:19-20)

I perceive this gift as the sign of a vocation in the potential. From the very moment when I was conceived, I was granted the potential of grace a prerequisite to every vocation. Time, circumstances, spiritual formation, humanistic and theological training, pain and illness, the loss of loved ones, all have served to arm me for victory for Christ over the forces of evil in my developing vocation.

I speak often of the topics "Called," "Being Called," and "To Surrender." This is because my surrendering to God allows the Father in heaven, through His Son, Jesus Christ, and through the dynamics of the Holy Spirit, to fashion me to be God's immediate channel of grace. Everything begins from God, is transmitted from God, works through God, is in God, and must end in God (*Per Ipsum, cum Ipso, et in Ipso*).

By nature, I am moved by anyone in need. I feel compelled, therefore, to give even more than might be requested. I remember an Irish panhandler who came to our rectory door. I was just about to leave for an errand when he came up to me. "Glory be to God," I quietly exclaimed to myself. Sizing him up, I knew how this meeting would end. "How may I help you, sir?" I asked as if I didn't know. That was all he needed to hear. That definitely was an invitation to unburden himself, yet he asked for no more than a bite and something to drink. With a smile I conducted him into the rectory and served him two sandwiches, a bowl of rich soup, coffee cake, and two cups of coffee. I not only shared this meal with him, but I was so scrupulously determined to help a beggar that when he left the rectory he walked out dressed in a black cashmere coat, black soft hat, and carrying two pairs of new black slacks and a suit.

Earlier, shortly after I had just been ordained and was serving in a Chicago parish, a poor Mexican family came to the rectory door seeking money for food. Being a Scalabrini missionary priest, I lacked the authority to give out money. I did the next-best thing to aid a hungry family. From the rectory kitchen's icebox I took out a frozen chicken. I discreetly and furtively wrapped the frozen chicken and some vegetables in a bag and sent the Mexican family homeward very happy.

I relate these incidents and events so that you may share my love for the sick and the poor. I hope, too, you will identify with my faults and failures as well as my strengths and achievements.

Though traditionally trained, I welcome the flexibility and freedom of contemporary religious practice. My roots of union with God are found not only in cell and classroom but also in the camp of life. Perhaps the best description of my present ministry is that I am an old pair of shoes polished up.

True, I have been called by God, and I pray that I remain His faithful link between the ancient Church and the present-day, contemporary Church. One must never forget that what was once new eventually in time becomes old; and that both old and new serve in their own age as stepping-stones for growth. As a link, I am perceived as proclaiming openly that there is no such thing as a charismatic Church in counterdistinction to the institutional Church. To see the two as separate or opposed entities is to accept a split in the Church of God. Indeed, to accept such a view is an attack on the very soul of Christ's Body, the Holy Spirit Himself. The Church is not an organization, but an organism bearing cells that grow with each age until reaching maturity in eternity.

Though I am considered a charismatic priest, owing to the gifts that function through me, I, like all responsible leaders, confirm Father Martin Tierney's concept (as stated in his book *The Hour of the Holy Spirit*, p. 9) that "The Charismatic Renewal is born to disappear. It is a mighty river flowing into the sea, which is the Church. When it reaches the sea and becomes completely mingled with it, it will lose its identity as a separate movement and the whole Church will be renewed."

Allegiance is to be given to God and to God alone. Loyalty to him must stem from the conviction that *nothing else will convert the world back to God* except the way of Jesus Christ. In the world in which we live, there is a deep spiritual hunger in the heart of man. This hunger will be satisfied by the very actions of Christ Himself: teaching, preaching, and healing.

In my own preaching, solidly founded in my faith and priestly function, I try to be clear, simple, and forceful. It is not what I say that touches people. The magnetic force of the message lies in the absolute trust and surrender that I teach about the Holy Spirit. It is His presence in renewed souls that *challenges Satan himself*. And when the Holy Spirit is present, healings and miracles result. Catholics, Protestants, Jews, believers, skeptics, and critics suddenly are enraptured in the presence of God's cloud, the "Shechinah, as it was called by the Hebrews of old. Suddenly, all begin to worship together. And the family of God becomes alive.

Some who have experienced this enfolding rapture have told me that I am a composite of Paul, who was constrained to preach Christ crucified, and Peter, who was called to walk to his Christ upon the water—dauntlessly, straightforwardly, directly. But it does not matter what I am called on to do; what matters is that I keep my eyes on the Christ before me, the God who beckons me onward. With eyes on Him, I need not falter or fear.

All men at some time in their lives receive a call to aspire to higher things, but many let the call go by. Nevertheless, to the honest person who searches for fulfillment before his God, Who is his beginning and his end, this call is ever being repeated and answered. Isaiah puts it unmistakably when he proclaims: "Strengthen all weary hands, steady all trembling knees and say to all faint hearts, 'Courage! Do not be afraid. Look, your God is coming . . . He is coming to save you.' Then the eyes of the blind shall be opened, the ears of the deaf unsealed, then the lame shall leap like a deer and the tongues of the dumb sing for joy." (Is. 35:3–6)

And so, therefore, in response to the public request that I take up my pen again to write anew some of the adventures of my soul with God, I find that I am revealing my journey with God to you. May these inner sentiments richly bless you in your own quest for holiness. May you return a response to the Master's cry not only by listening but by surrendering your total "you." May you, too, experience the healing compassion of the Master's love. May you, too, become a humble person serving God in the consciousness of your own nothingness.

It is my wish that, while it is only natural to admire gifts in others, one be encouraged "to get to know oneself": who one is, what one is, what gifts one has both natural and supernatural, and where one is going; and to get to know Who God is and to ask Him to bless these natural gifts. As we respond to the divine invitation to serve His call, may each one of us, both you and me, use for the first time, or use again freshly, all the charisms that He has endowed us with. May they become the extension of His person among all people. Perhaps you yourself can answer with your own personal response the question: "Why this man, O Lord?"

9

THE WOUNDED HEALER

Give the Earth to Christ
A little boy of heavenly birth,
but far from home today,
comes down to find His ball, the earth
that sin has cast away.
O comrades, let us one and all
join in to get Him back His ball.

"Give the Earth to Christ"
by John Bannister Tabb

Sweet Jesus! for how many ages hast Thou hung upon Thy Cross, and still men pass Thee by and regard Thee not, except to pierce anew Thy Sacred Heart. How often have I passed Thee by, heedless of Thy great sorrow, Thy many wounds, Thy infinite love! How often have I stood before Thee, not to comfort and console Thee, but to add to Thy sorrow, to deepen Thy wounds, to scorn Thy love!

Thou hast stretched forth Thy hands to comfort me, to raise me up, and I have taken those hands that might have struck me into Hell and have bent them back on the Cross and nailed them there,

* *To Jesus Forsaken,* Passionist Missionaries, Union City, N.J.

rigid and helpless. Yet I have but succeeded in engraving my name on Thy palms forever!

Thou hast loved me with an infinite love and I have taken advantage of that love to sin the more against Thee; yet my ingratitude has but pierced Thy Sacred Heart and forth upon me has flowed Thy Precious Blood. O sweet Jesus, let Thy Blood be upon me, not for a curse, but for a blessing. Lamb of God, Who takest away the sins of the world, have mercy on me!*

If a modern newspaper would turn its gaze back through the ages and centuries gone by and rest its interest upon the land of Palestine in the days in which a man called Jesus Christ, a Galilean, a Nazarean, lived, it would probably depict this Christ in a front-page article. Perhaps the writer of this newspaper column would write this story of the man of Galilee in the following fashion:

JESUS CHRIST, AS SEEN BY A
CONTEMPORARY

There has appeared in this our day, a man of great virtue, named Jesus Christ, who is yet living amongst us, and with the Gentiles is accepted as a prophet of truth, but his own disciples call him the Son of God. He raiseth the dead, and cureth all manner of diseases; a man of stature somewhat tall and comely, with a very reverend countenance; such as the beholder may both love and fear; his hair is of the color of a filbert, full ripe, and plain down to his ears, but from his ears downwards somewhat curled, and more orient of colour, waving about his shoulders. In the midst of his head goeth a seam or partition of hair, after the manner of the Nazarites; his forehead very smooth and plain; his face, nose and mouth so framed as nothing can be reprehended; his beard somewhat thick, agreeable to the hair of his head for colour, not of any great length, but forked in the middle; of an innocent and mature look; his eyes grey, clear and quick. In reproving, he is terrible; in admonishing, courteous and fair spoken, pleasant in speech, amidst gravity. It cannot be remembered that any have seen him laugh, but many have seen him weep. In proportion of body, well shaped and straight; his hands and arms most beauteous to behold; in speaking, very temperate, modest and wise; a man of singular virtue, surpassing the children of men.

PUBLIUS LENTULUS.†

† *The Joy of Words*, Chicago, Ill: J. G. Ferguson Pub. Co., 1960.

The last thing a person gives away to anyone is his heart: Time is expended and gifts are surrendered. God brought Himself into time, as revealed in the anointed Christ. The Christ gave away, as a prodigal son surrendering all, His earthly time to reveal the love of the Father; He offered as well the gift of forgiveness; moreover, He offered an invitation to a rebirth. To grasp the throbbing beat of the Wounded Healer, one must gaze upon Him Who had proclaimed that whatsoever would be raised up and would gaze upon Him would be healed. And so now we come to that moment in which a heart is truly tested in its love: *Crucifixion*—that is, how love, ardent and fiery as it may be in its initial stages, goes sour through its process of indifference and finishes in hate.

In the natural process of retaliation, a man who is exposed and surrendered to human crucifixions of life usually responds with curses and swearing and condemnation. He would even spit upon his executioners. But on that sad day in the history of man—if such a day could be called sad, for its effects upon man became good—the Son of God offers everything away: forgiveness, His holy mother, and now even His heart. In those agonizing hours, He offers the final drafts of His love; His heart is pierced. His precious blood, sacred blood, spurts out of gaping wounds and showers itself upon man. Every love call seeks a response. However, it is a real tragedy when such an invitation is declined by those who suffer—by the very ones whose pain Christ wants to heal through love. The tragedy of a broken heart is that love should be denied by those who are slaves of love and yet remain its stranger.

On the day that Christ died, three crosses were erected side by side. There is something of fascination in all stories of human sorrow. Each story of sorrow elicits a deep pathos within us. When we gaze upon the suffering of another, befogged with confusion over its reality, we seek to make its meaning sublime. But why turn our thoughts to any sorrow less sacred than that of the expiring Saviour, crowned with agony? As one gazes upon the Lord, other human sorrows pale to insignificance. Do not Zechariah 12:10 and John 19:37 adequately describe this pathos? "They will look on the one whom they have pierced; they will mourn for him as for an only son." Touched by His goodness when He walked the land, touched by His goodness as He walks into our daily lives, should we not touch Him as He hangs upon the cross for love of us? As Pascal says, Christ will be upon the cross forever until every man, woman and child comes to release Him from the cross.

Perhaps it would be good for us as we gaze upon the crucified love to proclaim: "Lord, it is good for us to be here!" As we cover our faces before that stupendous mystery of sorrow and as we bow our heads to ponder the Wounded Healer, we see that there was one alleviation to the great torture of this crucifixion. It was customary for wealthy ladies of that time to prepare a stupefying brew of sour wine, myrrh, and other ingredients now unknown when a crucifixion was to take place. The anodine, now being prepared, was sent as a full draft to each victim. If accepted by the crucified, it had the virtue to deaden pain and dull the mind.

Jesus tasted this potion when it was forced to His lips. He refused to drink it. He would meet the awful suffering with a clear mind. If the Cross is a symbol of the problem of pain, then the crucifix is its solution. The difference between the cross and the crucifix is the person of Christ being thrust upon it. As soon as Jesus mounted the cross, He revealed to the world how pain can be changed through love into a joyful sacrifice. His behavior on the cross was one of dignity and honor. It seemed to convey a message of how those who sow in tears can reap in joy. It seemed to cast a ray of hope to those who walked in darkness, now able to look unto the heavens and see the stars.

For many long hours, Jesus had hung there on the cross, suffering all the tortures of crucifixion and all the agonies of hell itself. "After this, Jesus knew that everything had now been completed, and to fulfill the Scripture perfectly he said: 'I am thirsty.' A jar full of vinegar stood there, so putting a sponge soaked in the vinegar on a hyssop stick they held it up to his mouth." (Jn. 19:28–29) On that infamous implement of Roman torture, the cross, Christ expounds His imperative, His intercession, His intervention, His interests, His isolation, His identification, His indemnity, His invincibility.

Each soul beneath the cross has its own description of what God is like. Studdert Kennedy, a parish priest and army chaplain during the First World War, while serving in France described and expressed in a striking and graphic manner an incident that had taken place as guns fired and bombs exploded along the trenches of that war-torn land. In his book *The Hardest Part*, Kennedy describes a conversation that took place in a base hospital between himself and another officer, who was slowly recovering from very serious wounds. The conversation turned to religion. In the face of his experience, in the anguish of a war-ravished body, the officer questioned Chaplain Kennedy: "What is God like?" Studdert Kennedy knew that his success or failure as a chaplain depended upon his answer. Choosing action rather than mere spoken word, he pointed out a crucifix which hung over the officer's bed and said: "Yes, I think I can tell you. God is like that." But the officer responded: "But I ask you, not what Jesus was like, but what God is like—God who willed His agony upon the cross, and who apparently wills the whole slaughter in this war. Jesus Christ I know and admire, but what is God almighty like? To me, He is still the unknown God." How would one answer such a question? How would you answer, yourself, with thousands of others like him who feel all that but cannot put their feeling into words? The only answer that I believe I can give within the pages of this chapter is that God, like His Son, Jesus, is despised and rejected by men.

St. Paul, great defender of the faith, staunch bearer and lover of Christ crucified, once came into Athens, the capital of Grecian culture, while it flourished in the heights of all its glory. Paul, though his eloquence was supreme in this incident, failed as he preached to ears that would not listen. Nevertheless, he said: "Men of Athens, I have seen for myself how extremely scrupulous you are in all religious matters, because I noticed, as I strolled around admiring your sacred monuments, that you had an altar inscribed: To an Unknown God. Well, the God whom I proclaim is in fact the one whom you already worship without knowing it." (Ac. 17:23) A masterpiece of art by Sigismund Goetze that hangs in a Boston gallery offers a dramatic re-creation. In this magnificent painting there is depicted before a stately, pillared temple an altar with the inscription: TO THE UNKNOWN GOD. A written description has been appropriately condensed by those wonderful priests of the Passionist Order, who themselves are professed to preach Christ crucified. The painting, described by human words, shows bound to this altar the living, shrinking, thorn-crowned Christ. His hair hangs down like a veil over His face to hide His shame and confusion. Before the naked person of Jesus a constant stream of humanity with all their selfish interests pass. Each one is utterly oblivious to the Victim on the cross. Each one stands beneath that cross with ingratitude.

As the observer studies the artist's portrayal, he can meditate as he sees a young lady of fashion, decked out in the most alluring style of the day. Flirting, she revels in the amorous glances of her dissipated escort. Neither can be distracted by the scourged Christ hanging alone, forsaken. There, too, stands a learned scientist, fascinated beyond fascination by his bubbling test tube. He is unaware of the infinite wisdom of God placed standing beside Him in public disgrace. The sport is there also. He strolls by, engrossed in the victory of his favorite horse. He has no time to notice the suffering Christ, Who can offer him the greatest victory, which is bought not by the wager of vice but by virtue of life.

At the base of the altar itself there are many onlookers to this portrait of man's life as it stands in relation to his God. The majority walk about Calvary's heights solely as spectators. First, among many, is to be seen a poor mother hugging her sickly child to her breasts. With tears that only pain can muster, she rests her weary limbs around this human creature enfolded within her maternal embrace. This forlorn outcast of humanity has turned her back on the bleeding Christ. Little does she know that even her repentance would have brought comfort to the Man of Sorrows overlooking her child as well as herself. A ragged newsboy is very busy in the hustle and bustle of hawking his extra: a scandalous divorce, mocking Christ's teaching on the indissolubility and sanctity of marriage. In the midst of the painting, at the base of the altar, where the crucified feet of Jesus are torturously seen, stands a pompous ecclesiastic dressed in fine robes. He struts by, so wrapped up in himself that he has no time for anyone else. Behind him comes the businessman. Scheming how he would be able to enlarge his fortune, he, too, fails to look upon Christ and looks instead to the world, with all its false promises, even to the cost of his soul, which is engaged in bad business.

Goetze paints even more significantly the time-serving politician—judge or counselor that he be—poring over his lawbooks. Blinded with pride, confused by graft, he cannot see clearly the purpose of his public service, nor does he see the solution of his case, unmistakably written in red upon the body of the Victim before him. As an adjunct to this incident, there, in the background, the observer finds a politician haranguing the crowd. He is so worried over his popularity that his soul would be the first thing he would barter for his reelection.

But there is one person who alleviates the anguish of the dying Christ. The power of grace touches this soul. Glancing aghast at the tortured Christ is a nurse, an angel of mercy. She is the only one in all that mob who has caught the tones of His pleading and the torture of His wounds. She is well trained. She is sensitive. Through hours of watching, tending the sufferings of men, she has discovered the answer to the mystery of human misery. The answer is love— love even to sacrifice. Love stronger than death! Love always wins!

Only he who has wounds can understand the wounds of another. There is nothing more touching and more impressive in Jesus than His tender compassion for the wounded and afflicted. Whoever reads through the gospels will find that two thirds of these New Testament scriptural passages relate events in which Jesus again and again makes use of His divine power of compassion over the human wounds of illness of spirit, soul and body. To relieve man's sufferings, Jesus would absorb unto Himself all the pain of those who would seek healing.

So very often by a word, a look, a touch, Jesus heals people: the blind man of Jericho, the servant of the Centurion, the infirm man at Bethsaida, the lepers, the paralytic at Capernaum. He even restores sight to the blind. He allows the deaf and the dumb to hear and speak. Luke depicts it clearly: "Everyone in the crowd was trying to touch him because power came out of him that cured them all." (Lk. 6:19)

All of us are called and summoned to soothe, ease, or heal our brothers and sisters. In so doing, we offer human compassion and concern to the very person of Christ, dwelling in humanity. Jesus impressed upon His disciples this immediate duty of sympathy and assistance to the sick and the suffering. He praised the charitable compassion of the Good Samaritan. He promised eternal reward to those who sympathize with the sick, the less fortunate: " 'Come, you whom my Father has blessed, take for your heritage the kingdom prepared for you since the foundation of the world. For I was hungry and you gave me food; I was thirsty and you gave me drink; I was a stranger and you made me welcome; naked and you clothed me, sick and you visited me, in prison and you came to see me.' Then the virtuous will say to him in reply, 'Lord, when did we see you hungry and feed you; or thirsty and give you drink? When did we see you a stranger and make you welcome; naked and clothe you;

sick or in prison and go to see you?' And the King will answer, 'I tell you solemnly, in so far as you did this to one of the least of these brothers of mine, you did it to me.'" (Mt. 25:34–40)

If a physician would be considered guilty of criminal neglect by refusing the assistance of his art to the human body, which must soon return to the dust of the earth from whence it came, how much more guilty would all of us be who are called Christians? To those who deny or neglect the cries of the sick, the hunger of the poor, or the wounds of the broken, the words of the Father spoken to the first murderer, Cain, will echo down the ages: "Yahweh asked Cain, 'Where is your brother Abel?' 'I do not know,' he replied. 'Am I my brother's guardian?' 'What have you done?' Yahweh asked. 'Listen to the sound of your brother's blood, crying out to me from the ground. Now be accursed and driven from the ground that has opened its mouth to receive your brother's blood at your hands. When you till the ground it shall no longer yield you any of its produce.'" (Gn. 4:9–12)

The cry of the Wounded Healer is the cry of a God man in search of a response of love from those whom He has loved unto the point of woundedness. His true cry is one of thirst: "I am thirsty." (Jn. 19:28) That significant cry is the cry of a God in search of souls: *Da Mihi animas*—"Give Me souls!" Loneliness is seldom thought of as a great hardship. Nothing makes suffering more piercing than loneliness. You and I are not strangers to this experience. You and I have felt, at times, that nobody really knows and nobody really cares about the veins of pain that circulate throughout our being. Loneliness can be compared to the last acid ingredient that instills into suffering its finest intensity in one explosive and thrusting crush: the death stroke of life's desolation.

"I thirst," He cried and, in that thirst, there He hangs as an outcast of heaven and earth. Endless minutes become hours that seem to have an eternal conviction and sentence. He searches the heavens for the presence of His Father, Who appears to have abandoned Him. With eyes that are bloodshot and now crusted with dried blood, He looks to the ground and gazes upon His mother. There John, the young and newly ordained priest, stands, faithful and loyal. Magdalene, too, is seen there, ever fulfilling the role that has given her perennial remembrance: a woman upon her knees in holy penitence. But His gaze shows more pain to His understanding than to His wounds: the rejection of the jeering mob. He now understands clearly that His rejection by His chosen race, by His scattered followers, would leave Him delivered into the hands of strangers, hanging there in public disgrace, laughed at by those He loves. And still His cry goes forth to heaven: "Father, forgive them; they do not know what they are doing." (Lk. 23:34)

Isaiah admonishes us:

Seek Yahweh [the Lord] while he is still to be found,
call to him while he is still near.
Let the wicked man abandon his way,
the evil man his thoughts.
Let him turn back to Yahweh [the Lord] who will take pity on him,
to our God who is rich in forgiving.

(Is. 55:6–7)

The Scriptures cry further, as they lament in their tenebrae of lamentation, how Christ came unto His own and His own received Him not. . . . Oh, that today you would hear His voice. Harden not your hearts. Peter himself in his First Letter, Chapter 2, verse 9, confirms as he states: ". . . you are a chosen race, a royal priesthood, a consecrated nation, a people set apart to sing the praises of God who called you out of darkness into his wonderful light . . . you were outside the mercy and now you have been given mercy."

To speak of Jesus as the Wounded Healer is to focus on His healing through His wounds and eventually by His death. In his Chapter 30, verse 17a Jeremiah elaborates on this concept when he states: "I will restore you to health and heal your wounds." The climax of healing is the death of Jesus Christ on Calvary. His death is the moment of freedom, the moment of truth. In the moment of the atrocity of His death, Jesus releases His spirit for the ultimate healing. One can feel His love, the pouring out of the sentiments of His heart so significant of His great desire, as He speaks at the Last Supper to His disciples: "I have longed to eat this passover with you before I suffer." (Lk. 22:15)

Through pain there is healing. Too often, because of the intensity and experience of pain, we do not recognize Him Who would heal us. Hosea 11:3 proclaims: "I took them in my arms; yet they have not understood that I was the one looking after them." How often the Lord speaks to us in His own apparent silence, in those moments of silence as when He slept in the bark of Peter with His apostles who were weathering the onslaught of the waves of the storm. His presence, though apparently silent, was there. Our Blessed Lord as the Wounded Healer absorbed our pains so as to transmit His healing love through His own divine blood transfusion. If we only could forget our own pains and look upon His pain, Who has absorbed us into Himself, we would forget ourselves and console Him. In that transference of our pain, our total selves, into His wounds, He Himself will, in turn, transfer His divine life into us.

As Christ would be the Wounded Healer, beckoning and receiving all that would be wounded seekers, so we who would experience the crucified love would turn from Jesus and be sent forth by Him to other wounded seekers. We all are wounded healers, especially after we have experienced His wounded love through our own wounded searchings. As Christ assumed the human nature to heal it, so it appears that at times in our failings, foibles, and follies, we also can become sensitized to man's sufferings: his wounds, his sensitivities, his anguish. By so doing, one becomes alive to another's pain. We can never hurt another human being when we love him or her.

The answer to our human weaknesses and to our apparent shortcomings, failures, sins, is not our bad will . . . but God's salvific plan to heal not only our own brokenness, but that of others, through the sensitivity experiences of our own humanity that enable us to recognize their pain and offer the human touch of healing. In our vulnerability we humbly assume the humanity of anguish in this other person. To heal is to understand the pain of another: to absorb it by our knowledge, to purify it by our service, to implore grace upon the world.

The message of the vision of the Cross and the cries of the voice that struck out not only over the area of Golgotha but across the ages of time up to this very moment is the message of a divine love that waits for you and me, for all mankind. The greatest love story in all the world is God's love for men. The Cross is not something that has happened; the crucifixion is something that is happening. It can be found in any place and at any hour in the human race. There are thousands of people who have burdens to be lifted, problems that need to be solved, and sin that needs to be forgiven. Thousands of persons who meander across their respective homelands at some moment in life come to a crossroad of decision. The world upon which we look is a mass of "broken body." The world to which we are called is one in which that brokenness comes into focus—the vision of Him who hung upon a cross. From that cross gush forth crimson drops of His precious blood: the gaping wounds of sin in need of healing.

The Cross of Jesus will unfold itself as the keystone of a triumphant life. When God's people gather around His Cross, respect His crucifixion inflicted upon Him by man's hate, God's love reigns more supreme as it washes each soul in that precious blood of the Lamb. Truly astounding things can happen in one's life! Once we learn the power of the blood of Jesus, once we perceive its use in coping with life's difficulties, then new horizons burst forth, spreading new rays of vision. Life with all its adventures—even those not yet experienced—becomes a new birth. If only one would behold the suffering of Jesus, such a one would appreciate the love of the Crucified. Nothing but His amazing love would have compelled Him to suffer for us in the abominable way that He did. Nothing has more power to bring a human being closer to divinity in the presence of Jesus than the consolation we return to Him Who was offering us condolence, forgiveness, and redemption through His passion. Lovers tend to be united. Therefore, if one would want to come closer to the heart of Jesus, let him immerse himself in the sufferings of the Master.

The love of the Crucified will forever take hold upon all men. The outstretched arms of Jesus on the cross are twenty centuries long. The love of the Crucified has power to bring a sinner to repentance. The love of the Wounded Healer inspires the human heart betrayed by life and its promises to a deeper love for Him. The concern of the Wounded Healer brings vision into reality, to responsibility. It causes one to see without denial that guilt is hurting the one we love, that sin can be clearly recognized for what it is. Helpless and tired, man no longer seeks an escape through neurotic or schizophrenic avenues. From his brokenness, from his woundedness, from life's very scars, he returns by a process of inscape to the reality of who he is, where he is going, and Who his God is. Countless people who have suddenly seen what Jesus endured for our sake have broken down in rivers of tears. Having looked upon such pain, people not only project their own anguish and identify with the

Wounded One but, released through a process of catharsis and ven-
tilation, they constructively return to adore the Lamb of God, Who
has given them blank sheets on which to write the concluding chapters of their own autobiography.

There is a mighty power lying hidden in the suffering of Jesus.
And those who follow Jesus, especially after having been healed in
their own wounds by His wound, return to this Master as disciples
of the Lord. Suddenly a bolt of light, a new presence, electrifies their
inner beings. With prudence tempering zeal, with foresight, prayer,
and love, they want to witness to the Lord and Saviour, Jesus. Their
ardent love compels them to do so. Those who have wept over their
sins, absorbed in the tomb of His humanity and purified by the person of His divinity, respond to Him with all their heart. Full of gratitude, they become sensitive to His call: "Come, take up [your]
Cross and follow me." (Mt. 16:24)

Love calls for love. In light of this, can one find the return of a
broken love to a wounded lover? Though many of us are broken, we
can still be loved. This truth is preserved in the Scriptures. The gospel records that two hardened criminals were crucified with Jesus.
The one on the left blasphemed Christ. But the other rebuked his
companion. The merciful forgiveness always present in the heart of
Jesus struck forth in the fullness of its power. It became grace touching the sin-hardened soul of that thief. The Master answered his
plea to remember him, and from Calvary's heights a thief and criminal whom people hated and wanted to forget was to have perennial
remembrance in the book of books. Jesus assured him: "Indeed, I
promise you . . . today you will be with me in paradise." (Lk.
23:43)

There have been many attempts to depict this mystery of divine
love. It has been done by many of us who have effectively experienced in our own lives the outpouring of Jesus' redemptive love. In
our own crying voice to be remembered, Jesus remembered us with a
heart of love, a heart of forgiveness, reconciliation, redemption,
righteousness, regeneration.

God is love. He came to earth with love. His whole vocation
sprung forth from love. He spent his days giving love. Love was His
whole existence. And now in this last moment on earth, as He hung
there between heaven and earth, He outpoured the fullness of His
love as Saviour and redeemer. Upon that penitent thief there must

have spurted from the wounds of the central figure, Jesus, some drops of that redemptive blood. Jesus, that day, was a success. He had come to save sinners by the shedding of His blood. That day, Jesus won the heart of the good thief in a mysterious manner. This Wounded Healer overwhelmed the penitent thief with mercy. The gaze of the Master impressed the thief, who in turn made a decision for the Lord Jesus Christ. A sinner became good as he himself offered compassionate understanding of the sufferings of the Master. He shouted to his brother on the cross to be still, for this just man hanging between them was not guilty of crime. He shouted further to his brother that they deserved this just punishment for their crimes.

A sinner, like the prodigal son, is a squanderer of his life, his talents, all that is within him, around him and of him. True contrition ushers one into a voyage of discovery: a discovery of oneself and a discovery of the God Who made him for a purpose. No excuses are needed. That thief who became good by touching the heart of the Master would offer no excuses for his irresponsible actions in life. All he had was a wounded seeker's heart. He recognized what he needed. It was there before him: THE WORD OF TRUTH.

All things lead to God, for God is the beginning and the end of all creation. God will utilize even the folly of man's deliberate choice of sin if that will bring man back to God. God will accept, because of the constancy of His love, any traveler on his own road to Damascus. Did He not do this with Saul of Tarsus? Did he not do this with Mary Magdalene, who proclaimed herself "a woman of sin"? As He dealt with her, did not His forgiving word lead her to new decisions, new choices? She who had squandered her natural, God-given gift of love inordinately, now, after the experience of Him Who was divine love, changed her object of earthly love to Him—as way, truth, and life. However, as a penitent woman, she followed the Lord to Calvary. And only as she knelt there did she realize Him to be what she had never recognized Him to be previously: the Wounded Healer, the Redeemer.

Is it not true that those who are truly penitent cry for assistance? The crucified love hears our cries, as He understands our cries through the cries that He himself echoed forth through His own humanity. As He spoke to the thief sweetly, as he spoke to Mary Magdalene, giving her new love, as He spoke with love to the

woman at the well, instilling in her new faith, as He spoke with
love to the woman caught in adultery, so He speaks to all mankind
the words that He uttered as He walked across the land: "And
when I am lifted up from the earth, I shall draw all men to myself." (Jn. 12:32)

The story of the Wounded Healer is a story that needs to be re-
told. A good story is always worth retelling. As children, after Dad
or Mother would read to us a fairy tale that was most pleasing,
would we not say with amazed eyes and smiling face: "Read it
again. Read it again. Read it again!" So the story of the Wounded
Healer is the narration of a God Who sent His Son into an arena of
human conflict to be scarred and wounded, put to crucifixion and to
death. It is the story of Him Who was wounded that He might
heal. It is the story of Him Who died, was buried, arose from the
dead retaining His scars as a victorious warrior overpowering and destroying that which would lead to a tomb of death.

As long as man has breath to breathe and life to live, he will be
confronted by a host of forces that will either enrich him or deper-
sonalize him. But blessed is that person who will look up to the
heavens through the vista of Calvary's cross and see a loving Father
embracing him through the love of His Son, Jesus Christ. Caryll
Houselander adequately ascribes to Christ, as well as to His followers, these attributes when he says that some people in life learn
to love the whole world through the love of God; for them, the way
of sacrifice is direct and informed with joy. Others learn to love God
through loving one another . . . the heart that has been exchanged
for Christ's heart radiates from the love of its own children to all
the children of God, because now it cannot fail to love the heavenly
Father Himself *as Christ loves him.*

With a heart of love uniting itself to the heart of Him, we surrender to the language of verse:

> *O Christ, upon Thy Cross I set my gaze.*
> *The vision of Thy wounds deep within me seep.*
> *O Christ, upon Thy Cross I set my gaze.*
> *Speak to me words of Thy forgiving embrace.*
>
> R.D.O.

May the Cross of Christ ever continue to unveil its shining light
like the many facets of a diamond. But may one special facet of that

gleaming Cross stand out most prominently. Let each man who is drawn to healing, either to be healed or to heal, observe not as a spectator but as a soul saved by grace. As he kneels before the sacred image of the crucified humanity of Jesus Christ, let him contemplate *the love of the man divine Who bore the cross upon His back.*

10

HIS CROSS/HIS PRAYER

*If you want to know about God,
there is only one way to do it: Get
down on your knees. The man who
thinks only of himself says prayers
of petition; he who thinks of his
neighbor says prayers of intercession; he who thinks only of loving
and serving God says prayers of
abandonment to God's will, and
that is the prayer of the saints.*

ARCHBISHOP FULTON J. SHEEN

All who pray for others enter thereby into a holy fellowship of
intercession.

R.D.O.

As you read and meditate upon this chapter, you will have tapped
the source of my life and its mission. It is also the power of any authentically blessed individual who goes forth into the arena of the
world as a channel of God. *This is the power of prayer.* There is no
substitute for genuine conversation with God, and God in turn with

His created soul. Prayer must have its priority. It is as essential to us as water for a plant.

The tremendous success of a person's life, as related to any phase of his existence, derives from the fact that such an individual has entered into the deep recesses of his soul. Touched by prayer, a man of significance comes forth not because of his or her own energy but because of Him Who has permeated every fiber of existence with His abiding strength. Somewhere, I once read that the secret of any successful crusade for souls rests in the truth that we are all one in that Mystical Body of which Christ is the Head. Whatever good we do has an effect on the other members. It produces a spread of sanctity comparable to the chain reaction of a single atom splitting up and then having an effect on another atom as it in turn splits up and then another and another. It does so millions and millions of times over until each affecting the other finalizes in a mighty explosion.

And so, with the power of prayer, a human being who soaks his or her daily life in prayer nourishes the Mystical Body with a tremendous impact of the total sanctity of each member. The influence of that prayer uttered from a soul in union with God becomes so supernaturally dynamic that it bears the power to cover the whole face of the earth with God's compassionate, healing love. A person need not go into the mission fields or on evangelistic crusades to preach stimulating and restorative sermons. One just needs simply to rest with the thoughts of the Lord that are triggered by man's intercessory prayer. This is being an apostle through prayer. The power, because of its source, is infinite; its effects upon the world are immense.

It has also been reflected upon and said often by humble evangelists that spiritual renewals and evangelistic success are not the product of gifted personages. Neither do the powers of natural organizations, with all their skills and personnel, effect the salvation of humanity. But it is because the God of all graces showers down upon the human race countless blessings in response to "believing prayer."

Among Christians as they assemble together forming one body, *prayer is primary*. Among the charismatic groups, the gifts that reign realistically among them fulfill their own purpose—namely, the building up of the other members. Possessing, therefore, community-oriented gifts, the finest of all is that of *intercessory prayer*. This power of intercession means a coming between. Between God and those who justly deserve God's chastizing hand are heard the cries and pleas of the INTERCESSOR.

The Lord's injunction to pray is very forceful. Isaiah (59:16) zealously utters forth: "And He saw that there was no man, and was astonished that there was no one to intercede." Again, encouragingly, we read from 1 John 5:14, 15: "We are quite confident that if we ask him for anything, and it is in accordance with his will, he will hear us; and, knowing that whatever we may ask, he hears us, we know that we have already been granted what we asked of him."

Prayer is the beginning of all that is good in man. Therefore, it is of inestimable value to become familiar with prayer, to value it greatly, to love it, and to use it rightly and zealously. We are able to use it both here on earth and in eternity. Before the august throne of God our prayers can *adore* Him as we praise God for Who and What He is. Before His throne, the angels present to Him our thanksgivings for all the wonders He has given to us. How often people speak to us, humbly and hopefully, pleading with us to pray for them by imploring God to understand their errors performed through human weaknesses! In desperate search of heavenly blessings, these beseeching human beings approach another human person, believing that God would hear more readily the prayerful concern of an intercessor. We all have the obligation to intercede for others, that hindrances affecting positive fellowship and growth be eradicated. Like Christ, we assume the wounds of the world and we present them to the throne above.

We are encouraged to ask about anything and everything. God keeps His promises, for did He not say that if we asked anything in His name He would grant it? And because we believe in His word, we approach the throne to intercede and to ask on behalf of others. How enriching is the life and experience of prayer! St. John Vianney, the parish priest of Ars, once stated: "A soul in union with God through prayer is always in springtime." St. Paul, in his First Letter to Timothy, Chapter 2, verses 1 and 8, synthesizes these acts of prayer when he states: "My advice is that, first of all, there should be prayers offered for everyone—petitions, intercessions and thanksgiving. . . . I want the men to lift their hands up reverently in prayer, with no anger or argument."

Whenever one receives a gift, one can do with that gift whatever one wishes. One can either put it aside or enrich it, embellish it to further maturity. Praying is a gift; but at the same time it is also an art that must be learned by everyone. The Holy Spirit is the teacher in prayer. His instructions come either directly or through others. As He speaks to us through Scriptures, we see the importance and predominance of prayer. Meditating upon its values unravels profound insights. St. Teresa of Ávila discerned its substance when she prayed: "From foolish devotions may God deliver us!"

St. Alphonsus Liguori wrote a little booklet entitled *Gran Mezzo Della Preghiera.* In its Introduction, the saintly Bishop of Agata dei Goti says: "I have published several spiritual works, but in my estimation this little pamphlet on prayer is by far the most useful, because prayer is a means necessary and infallible in order to attain eternal salvation, and all the graces we need to obtain it. If it would be possible I would have many copies of this booklet, as many as are the faithful living on earth and I would give one to each of them so that everybody would understand the necessity that we all have to pray in order to be saved." In the very first chapter of this booklet the great Doctor of the Church proves that prayer is necessary (*"necessitate medii"*) in order to save our souls.

Jesus Himself was a "personification" of prayer. Every moment of His earthly life was imbued with, and expressed itself in, prayer. Who can accurately describe the life of prayer that Jesus must have spent there in the seclusion of Galilee? His daily labor as Joseph the carpenter's son was certainly mingled and sanctified with prayer. Even during His public life, which was so short, He gave much of His time to prayer. His initial program of evangelizing found Him, immediately after His submission to John's baptism, going into the desert to be alone with Himself and with His Father. In the confines of the desert experience, His prayer life was enriched by prayer's concomitant grace: fasting. How often His apostles witnessed their Master at prayer, in the early hours of the morning as well as in the last moments of the night. They were astonished and awestruck at His teachings and miracles; but in the final analysis, they recognized that the source of His power lay in those innersanctum moments of prayer. They were so impressed with Him that as they followed Him they wanted all the more to be like their Master. They needed His source of life. The scriptural narrative is so impellingly didactic. It offers with abundant wealth the answers to their honest plea: *Domine, doce nos orare*—"Lord, teach us how to pray": "Now once he was in a certain place praying, and when He had finished one of his disciples said, 'Lord, teach us to pray, just as John taught his disciples.' He said to them, 'Say this when you pray:

> Father, may your name be held holy,
> Your kingdom come:
> give us each day our daily bread,
> and forgive us our sins,
> for we ourselves forgive each one who is in debt to us.
> And do not put us to the test.' " (Lk. 11:1–4)

Before any public behavior or presentation, He was wont to offer that moment-to-come to His Father's glory. How often He indicated to the crowds that He and the Father were one and that all glory should be given to the Father! A perfect example of this was seen by those who witnessed the raising of Lazarus from the grave. How even more impressive was the splendor of prayer when Jesus taught Peter, James, and John a very special lesson as He Himself allowed His selected ones to experience true ecstatic prayer in the sparkling illumination of the Transfiguration! It was the first time that they had experienced this extraordinary form of slaying in the spirit. As they witnessed their Master transformed and raised on high, they themselves were radiant in the illuminating blaze of ecstasy: Their external senses were suspended; their human souls lost contact with the external world; their willpower had no control to terminate this state. What a privileged ecstasy!

Every page of the sacred writers, as they tell His story, is richly replete with this God-man at prayer. When the end of His life came and the cross of Calvary threw its shadow over Him, He prepared for it by the finest preparation He could bring to Gethsemane. *That was His supreme hour!* From that cross He would hang between God and man, interceding on behalf of humanity's needs. We are not surprised, therefore, after considering the action of Our Blessed Saviour, to hear Him insisting again and again on the importance of prayer: *"Oportet semper orare et numquam deficere."* Then He told them a parable about the need to pray continually and never lose heart. Again He states: *"Petite et accipietis, quaerite et invenietis, pulsate et aperietur vobis"*—Ask and it shall be given to you. For everyone who asks receives, and who seeks finds, and to him who knocks it is opened. Matthew records the Master as saying: "*Vigilate et orare ut non intretis in tentationem*"—"You should be awake, and praying not to be put to the test." (Mt. 26:41)

Following the example of the Divine Master and Model, all the saints, without exception, have been persons of prayer. Whether contemplative or given to active life, their main concern was *prayer*. They sacrificed everything in favor of prayer, because they knew very well that without prayer they could do nothing. We are not surprised to hear that they spent four or five hours in prayer every day, and for the rest of the day they were interiorly recollected, they were walking constantly in the divine presence of God.

To pray is the simplest thing on earth and in human life. It is essentially simple just because it is so necessary. We can see in nature that things that are most needed are the most common, the most simple: water, bread, air. It is the same in the supernatural order: Of all the sacraments, the one necessary for all in order to be saved is baptism. See how Jesus instituted it: The matter is the most common element that can be found everywhere, the form is the simplest: In case of necessity anyone can be the minister, even a person in the state of mortal sin or a non-Catholic, even a pagan. To pray needs no eloquence, no learning, no money, no earthly recommendation. It doesn't even require any special feeling or devotion. Sensible consolation in prayer is only an accompaniment and quite a secondary one. Sweetness in its exercise does not in the least depend upon us. God gives it, and we should receive it thankfully.

In order to pray, we need only to know God and ourselves, to understand Who He is and who we are, to realize how immeasurable is God's fatherly goodness and how unfathomable our own misery. Prayer, essentially, consists in the elevation of the heart and mind to God, to glorify Him and seek His blessings. From this we understand that faith and the catechism are the only knowledge we need bring to prayer. For prayer itself, only a few thoughts of the mind are requisite, the fewer the better: few desires of the heart and few words. But the words must spring from the heart, or else there is no prayer. God is ever ready to give His grace, and He gives it to each and all. "And if you have faith, everything you ask for in prayer you will receive." (Mt. 21:22) "Whatever you ask for in my name I will do." (Jn. 14:13)

To pray is simply to speak with God, to converse with Him by adoration, praise, thanksgiving, petition, and self-deprecation. Some say that prayer is a report we present to our good God or an audience He grants us. In an altogether too formal manner does this express the truth. Let us think of prayer as a familiar conversation with a good and kindly man. We trust him, we speak together of the most important things, quite plainly and often without emotion. All that matters is that we speak honestly and earnestly.

God has permitted us to pray, and so prayer is our right. He has commanded us to pray, and so prayer is our duty. Since all the elements of our being ultimately come from God, the only source of goodness and being, it is from Him that we must seek the good things that we want both in the natural and in the supernatural orders. It is true that God, in His love, has made provision for the good things that we need; nonetheless, our petitions to Him, implicit or explicit, are requested for these reasons: to acknowledge that we must ultimately receive everything from Him. "Give us each day our daily bread." (Lk. 11:3) And it can well be that God's eternal providence has decreed this benefit to us only in dependence on the prayer that He foresaw we would say. Thus prayer is not intended to change the changeless God but, rather, to fulfill the necessary law of His eternal knowledge and providence. This attitude of dependence on God as expressed in prayer is the principal form of the spirit of faith that Our Divine Redeemer so constantly demanded of those whom He cured, and of those who followed Him. It is this spirit of prayerful faith that explains the power of the saints. No one could be more conscious of his own limitations, no one more startling in audacity, than the saint in his consciousness of his access to God's omnipotence by prayer.

All of us, at one time or another, have been approached by other human beings seeking our interest in them by having us pray for them. These persons are seeking presence—the presence of another human being who will love them and not reject them, who will take their concerns to his own heart, who will assume their human pain and transform it through prayer into a hopeful, better expectation. The person in between is an *intercessor*. Once the cries and the anguish are received, he who assumes these petitions stands between the Almighty God above and the finite creature below as one who intends to pray for others with power, love, and understanding. How beautifully sensitive is the power of intercessory prayer! It is so much like a creative encounter with God. Fundamentally it undergoes an experience of real communion in which God and mind become one. Once again, God is portrayed as Francis Thompson's Hound of Heaven in search of the human soul that has groped arduously and anguishedly:

> I fled Him, down the nights and down the days;
> I fled Him, down the arches of the years;
> I fled Him, down the labyrinthine ways
>   Of my own mind; and in the midst of tears
> I hid from Him, and under running laughter.
>   Up vistaed hopes I sped;
>   And shot, precipitated,
> Adown Titanic glooms of chasmèd fears,
> From those strong Feet that followed, followed after. . . .
> (For, though I knew His love Who followèd,
> Yet was I sore adread
> Lest, having Him, I must have naught beside) . . .
>   Still with unhurrying chase,
>   And unperturbèd pace,
> Deliberate speed, majestic instancy,
>   Came on the following Feet,
>   And a Voice above their beat—
> "Naught shelters thee, who wilt not shelter Me."
> "[But come now, take my hand,] I am He Whom thou seekest!"

F. THOMPSON, The Hound of Heaven (19th cent.)

Intercessory prayer is primarily asking the Father to care for another because God cares for this person as well as do we. Enclosed within the prayer of intercession lies the dimension of love for another human. No man remains a stranger to this type of prayer. As the little boy carrying the other little fellow on his shoulders would say: "He ain't heavy, Father, he's my brother," so the intercessor carries upon his wings of prayer the needs of another human being.

In speaking to Heaven about another human soul, the intercessor converses with the Father in Jesus' name. With Jesus as the Redeemer, the intercessor through Christ implores the power of the Holy Spirit to bring about the kingdom. The heavens with their abundant graces are opened just because someone asked, just because someone had the time and the concern to unite with present petitions. As one lives the life of intercession by assuming the other person's needs, one "feels the burden" of the Lord for this specific person or need. The joy of this prayer is that we are praying with the Lord, through the Lord, and for the Lord's broken body, still wounded in the world.

Intercession may appear to be very sacrificial and time-consuming as well as truly committing. But it must be done. God has asked man to intercede for another. It is part of the Father's plan for bringing about His kingdom. It is the way that He desires us to ask for graces. The effect of this form of praying is realistic: When we receive the grace, we know that it is truly a gift from God. It shows our dependency upon Our Heavenly Father, and so we therefore render Him gratitude and glory. The greatest intercessor was Jesus Christ. As He hung there on that cross, He made His finest plea: "Father, forgive them; they do not know what they are doing." (Lk. 23:34)

With every passing moment, the sufferings of our crucified Lord became more terrible. Both His body and His soul were in the deepest torment. His body was now numb and listless. And while His spirit bore this torture, a burning heat was raging in His body. His lips were parched and dry. The saliva was sticky. The flowing blood from adjacent wounds was all that seemed to quench His thirst. Each taste of it made Him realize that He was there upon that cross. It was His duty to suffer this atrocity as a victim lamb. It was His understanding and love *to intercede* before heaven and earth, before God and man. Through this intercessory oblation, Jesus on the cross was beating a new heart into Christian religion. He gave life to Christian faith by the way He lived, prayed, and died.

When one speaks of the cross, one cannot help but think of Jesus, Who was cast upon it. When one thinks of Jesus on the cross, one cannot help but listen to *His prayer* uttering forth seven thoughts of healing love. As He was hanging upon that cross, he was interceding. As He was interceding, every drop of His tortured being was a healing transfusion of redemptive love. Those beneath the cross hated Him, so could not perceive the mystery of this cross—no one, that is, but Mary, John, Magdalene, and a few loyal friends. Hatred can cause eyes to be blind especially when prejudice and hardness precede. As His enemies cursed Him and derided Him, they could not perceive that as they killed Him, He was giving them life; that as they wounded Him, He was imparting healing. How very prophetic was Hosea (11:3): "I took them in my arms; yet they have not understood that I was the one looking after them."

When one speaks of the Crucifixion, one spontaneously draws closer to that Deicide incident. Moreover, the sounds of a dying man in excruciation are impressive, as they are unforgettable. As strange and as out of the ordinary as they may be, nevertheless, each message flowing forth from those anguished cries is absolutely different and distinctive, as it is very personal.

And so it was with the Divine Intercessor. Man's love had gone sour. Love's arrows became hateful spears piercing Him, Who became the Wounded Healer. Invectives burst forth from lips that should have prayed for forgiveness. That day, which became known as Good Friday, became a memorial day never possible to be forgotten. Indescribable wildness rampaged with its boisterous passion for blood and death.

Because Jesus remained faithful to that Cross, because His utterances spoke of intercession, many souls have been saved. Down to our days, an infinite number have found consolation in suffering; many hearts, hardened by sin, were softened and changed, considering the tears and the streams of blood shed by Our Lord. To many, the cross of the wounded Intercessor has become a victorious sword in the conflict of life. Many more have found peace, and rest for their own wounds. The Cross of Jesus has become truly a staff on the road to eternity, a tree of life for blossoming of new virtue. St. Augustine calls the passion of Jesus an altar upon which Our Lord offered Himself for our salvation. He calls the Cross of Jesus a pulpit from whence the wounded Christ not only instructs us in the virtues of obedience, love, humility, meekness, patience, and resignation, but from whence Jesus stands before God and man as Intercessor. *His cross became the pulpit for his prayer.*

God wants His world healed. God has sent His Son, Jesus, to heal it. Let us praise the Lord, Who has enriched the world with willing souls who are ready to dedicate themselves for the building up of His people and for the service of humanity. Let us offer gratitude to the Lord, Who continues to send out His call. The Lord calls for intercessors. He seeks generous lives who are substantially authentic in their loyalty to Him in spite of their weaknesses. He invites unto

Himself those persons sufficiently humble in the graces He has imparted to them. He invites men and women, children and teenagers, the young and the elderly, the sick and the healthy—all mankind— to respond to the call of intercession.

The way to God's power is through prayer. Prayer can do all things that God can do . . . and God wills that all things be accomplished through prayer/union with Him. The most deceiving plot of the devil is to keep people off their knees. Christ Jesus told us: "The harvest is rich but the laborers are few, so ask the Lord of the harvest to send laborers to his harvest." (Mt. 9:38) At this command of Jesus, each one of us should go forth as a center of spiritual radiation. Our intercessory prayer can spread out and continue in the churches, communities, families, the hearts of the faithful. Our Lord, Who commanded this form of concerned prayer for laborers, has also personally called those laborers. The words of His call are preserved in the treasure of the gospel: "Follow me and I will make you fishers of men." (Mt. 4:19) Those of us who are called to intercede should likewise make His call heard by others. In so doing we become like those atoms I spoke about in the beginning of this chapter: One splits and another splits, until there is had a tremendous explosion. The people of God have a right to His call to renewal.

Moreover, our intercessory prayer must be truly global. Let our prayer be a wholehearted prayer. Our minds must be open to God's global love for all His children. This means that we must transcend the boundaries of each local area, nation, religious community, and rite. Our life is a gift of God. We must do something good with it, using it for serving the broken body the Church, the broken body of society, broken humanity in all its enslavements. Everyone has the duty to pray. Everyone has the duty to cooperate in the building up of the Mystical Body of Christ. People who pray can constitute a bond with each other as community. The community relationship will flourish into all forms of social and ecclesial betterment. But the foundation of this must be that of prayer.

As we look about the world in which we live, we see that science has taught us how to do many things, including how to harness the power of the atom. But how very few of us have learned how to develop fully the tremendous power of prayer! We seem not to have learned that a man is more powerful on his knees than behind the

most powerful weapons that can be developed. We should make it
our everyday duty, as a vital element in our daily existence, to pray.
To pray in whatever we do, wherever we may go; to pray so as to
seek the presence of God. To pray that many confused souls may
not be strangers to His ways but may find His presence.

To be a genuine intercessor, one must know or learn how to really
pray. And one of the first lessons is *silence*. Silence inspires decision.
This sentence is worth repeating, because decision is inspired by silence. Silence brings us into ourselves. It offers us the voyage of the
within, a journey of discovery into our spiritual, mental and moral
security. It clarifies our meaning and goal of life. As we make that
journey within, there is no longer any room for escapism as a fleeing
from something: as a substitute for not fulfilling our duties. Silence
introduces the power of prayer into our lives so that we respond to
God and man with truthfulness and honesty and with responsible
service. Yes, silence does lead to decision. Silence does have a voice!

A place of *solitude* is another important factor for him who
wishes to pray. It is interesting to note that in all walks of life we
see that when all is said and done, *much more is said than done*.
Never before did the world talk as much as it does in our modern
day. The host of mass communication media have influenced conversation beyond its reasonable use. It has served as an outlet for dissipation. Never before has there been such a barrage of talk. Eventually man cries for solitude. The tension of communication is too
great and strenuous. Should not a place be found to offer opportunities for prayer with oneself, with one's God, to intercede for the
world? Does not everyone search out those quiet moments when
thoughtlessness becomes thoughtfulness through the power of
prayer?

Many people speak only to be heard. Very few people know how
to retreat into themselves so as to experience the splendor of a
"requiem of silent communication" between their God and their
souls. The call to worship makes no loud noises. Yet, all of us are
bound to worship the Almighty with our thoughts, with our actions,
our behavior, our personalities, our vocations. How can we be ener-
gized to fulfill our daily responsibilities to God, to ourselves, to our
fellow men, unless we stop to reflect and to pray? No one can know
his own soul or his journey in life; no one can answer the summons

to abide in joy unless the still, peaceful voice of God is heard from within.

Amid circles of conversation today, there is frequently heard the statement that God is dead. The truth of the matter is that God is silent due to the death of our ears, our deafness to His voice. Our language, with its multiple forms of communication, frequently renders itself a camouflage. It conceals our real thoughts, and we fail to heed the admonition of Shakespeare, "To thine own self be true." But a retreat into silence produces honest conversation with truth, and the truth discovered sets us at liberty "to be." By comparison we could say that just as the body needs rest and sleep from its strenuous toil and strain, so does the soul require that special quiet solitude that offers openness to "another presence," the person of God.

It is often recognized when we look about the world in which we live that man is like the Temple of Jerusalem, which was made up of three courts. There was the outer court, for the gentiles, who came in to watch and who cared little for the great mysteries being enacted in the interior part of the Temple. Next, there was a sanctuary, or the holy place where only the Hebrew worshipers might gather. Finally, there was the Holy of Holies, into whose secluded chamber only the high priest entered—alone and but once a year. So man lives in three courts, we could say. Outside is the court of the world, with its business, its humdrum routine, its commercial frenzy, its social encounters, its personal involvements. Next is the holy place, where man walks with those who share his beliefs, be they political, economic, or religious, and where he suffers great perplexities and stress. Sometimes the tremendous anxieties he encounters in the holy place destroy him. Finally, there is the Holy of Holies, where God dwells, where in guarded reticence secrets pass between his soul and his God.

The silence that leads to decision is nothing else but prayer. When we retreat from the hustle and bustle of life's encounters and activities to place ourselves in the presence of Almighty God, a dynamic interaction results. This mutual interplay is called dialogue, or conversation. And while dialogue helps discussion, silence gives birth to decision. It is important to remember that. Conversation presents points of view; but it is through silence that one surrenders to magnanimous conviction.

A daily journey with prayer can be very exciting. If you would allow divine grace to supernaturalize your psychological methods, you could find a tremendous amount of peace of mind and strength of soul. The following simple steps might be interesting for you, as they can be helpful to the development of your prayer life. They are very unpretentious, but powerful in their influence. They may assist you, as they have been a constant tool all through my prayer life.

First, set aside by daily resolution an hour a day for silence in which to look into yourself as you would gaze into a mirror. To do this will also create an openness to inspiration from without. The world with all its beauty as created by God will suddenly be seen with a new vision. Everything will have its own place and its own purpose. We will find new insights to the universe, to its science, to the human circumstances that become so much a part of our existence. A truly divine purpose will instill our understanding about the places we go, the places we dwell in, the things we are summoned to act upon, the people we meet. Insight and discovery will untangle the countless perplexities of our divergent behaviors. We can even make a list of our actions. In response to each item of behavior, we can list the "why's." Interestingly enough, you will see that all the actions listed can be attributed to two or maybe three dominant factors. These factors can then be improved by the appropriate virtue.

God is faithful to us. A human love encounter easily can decline with time; but divine love does not. Neither theological knowledge nor social action alone is enough to keep us in love with Christ unless both are preceded by a personal encounter with Him. Christ must be felt first. Christ is constantly inviting us to come to Him, that He may take us to the Father. He brings us to Himself through the ups and downs, through the tear-stained sacrifices of life, through the joys and pains that are parceled in this life. As its remedy, He invites us to converse with Him, to ask for such things as are of major or minor concern, and to experience the ineffable blessing of "fellowship" with Him. If you and I were to place ourselves before the brilliantly flaming sun, we would both be radiant in the glow of its light. There, basking in that illumination, we sit quietly and humbly in His presence, like a body exposing itself before the sun to absorb its rays. It is exactly at this point that true prayer springs forth. *God speaks to us, and we listen!*

Second, a good practice is to write down the inspirations derived from these moments of encounter with God and self. Within these notebooks are recorded the precious contents flowing from the "prayer book" of your heart. Varied are the sentiments: aspirations, regrets, one's yearnings, failures, hopes, and fears; reflections from other human hearts, retreat experiences, the joys of life, the pains, along with the divine graces that elevate them into stepping-stones of perseverance. The art of writing has a potential of aiding one to place in balance one's thoughts and experiences. It facilitates objective consideration through silence as one verges toward "decision." Our jottings in our notebooks continue to reiterate to ourselves that when God gives grace, we can believe; when He withdraws grace, we cannot believe. God's will is that we harvest the fruits of our encounters with life, our God, our fellowships, and with ourselves. Harvest time lasts only a few weeks. The harvest does not wait for anybody. One either gathers it or loses it. Our consciousness should assist us to be careful that the time of opportunity does not pass us by. "The harvest is over, summer at an end, and we have not been saved." (Jr. 8:20)

Third, let nothing interfere with this period of silence. Do it not because other persons are doing it. Do not perform it as a spiritless duty. Do not even fulfill it as an end in itself. But do it because God has granted this priceless privilege to come into His presence, to covenant with Him. The busier you are, the more you need this hour. By faith and discipline you can become loyal in this practice. Your life will be rich. You will know who you are, you will know where you are going, and you will know Who your God is.

Fourth, perform this hour with meditation, that you may order yourself into two directions. The first is to God, adoring Him in the purest kind of prayer, because it is all for God. There is nothing in it for you. As you worship Him, you cannot help but love Him for Himself. He is Greatness, Wisdom, Holiness, Glory, Grace, Power, Knowledge, Love. He is Himself. As you continue to be specific in your adoration and gratitude to Him, His voice will respond rapidly and very emphatically that *He loves you*. The assurance of His presence and His love will then lead you to community concerns. Therein the world becomes your parish. You can touch it through the power of intercessory prayer. Through your own encounter with Divinity you were getting light from the sun while still walking on the earth. And so your personal prayer must now radiate its own illumination to others, who may still be in search of the Light. You have allowed the Holy Spirit to have His way with you, fixing no rules to your hour of quiet with Him—as there are no fixed rules for loving. So now allow that Holy Spirit to utilize you to provide a bridge for Him to others.

What a powerful weapon God granted us when He gave us the grace to utilize the prayer of intercession. Ask for others. Stand in for others such as missionaries, foreign lands, our country, the church, students, the young and the old, the sick and the dying. Pray and intercede for friends and enemies. Pray and intercede for the people of many lands who have yet to hear about Jesus.

Intercessory prayer is so powerful that the Scriptures record pages of interesting events. Let's journey through a few of them:

Genesis 19:17–21 reads: "As they were leading him out they said, "Run for your life. Neither look behind you nor stop anywhere on the plain. Make for the hills if you would not be overwhelmed." "No, I beg you, my lord," Lot said to them, "your servant has won your favor and you have shown great kindness to me in saving my life. But I could not reach the hills before this calamity overtook me, and death with it. The town over there is near enough to flee to, and is a little one. Let me make for that—is it not little?—and my life will be saved!"

Here the Lord is about to destroy Sodom and Gomorrah. He answers Lot, "I grant you this favor too, and will not destroy the town you speak of." The town was named Zoar. As the sun rose over the land and Lot entered Zoar, Yahweh rained brimstone and fire on Sodom and Gomorrah. He destroyed these towns with all their inhabitants and everything that grew there.

God listened to Lot's prayer. Lot *interceded*.

In Exodus 32:11–14 we find: "But Moses pleaded with Yahweh his God. "Yahweh," he said, "why should your wrath blaze out against this people of yours whom you brought out of the land of Egypt with arm outstretched and mighty hand? Why let the Egyptians say, "Ah, it was in treachery that he brought them out, to do them to death in the mountains and wipe them off the face of the earth"? Leave your burning wrath; relent and do not bring this disaster on your people. Remember Abraham, Isaac and Jacob, your servants to whom by your own self you swore and made this promise: "I will make your offspring as many as the stars of heaven, and all this land which I promised I will give to your descendants, and it shall be their heritage for ever." So Yahweh relented and did not bring on his people the disaster he had threatened."

Here again we have Moses asking God to *intercede* for the people despite their idolatry. All sin is nothing but idolatry, whether we realize it or not. When we turn for gratification to people or things, we are making little gods of them. That is where the sin is. You turn away from God, you turn away from the power that is the only important one. Moses asks God not to be angry with his people. Many of the misfortunes in the country today are happening because there is no one to enter into his own heart, his own holiness, in order to *intercede*.

In 1 Timothy 2, Paul tells Timothy to pray for everyone, which includes sinners. And Isaiah 53:12 talks about praying all the time for sinners. Here we see the great pattern set by Jesus—our model for intercessory prayer. We all must follow that pattern if we are to make our land a holy one.

What are the four ways that Jesus served as the great Intercessor? They are the things Jesus did on the cross:

—He poured out his blood—a life-giving element;
—He was "numbered among the transgressors" to heal them;
—He bore our sins—and so we are asked to bear the burdens of our brothers and sisters;
—He made intercession for His crucifiers; He forgave them; He loved *them* to the very end.

Simply put, then, intercession is nothing else but asking the Father in the name of Jesus for the power of the Holy Spirit. For what purpose? To bring about the kingdom. What is that kingdom? Salvation . . . and health . . . and healing. This is real *liberation*.

Therefore, I beg you to look for the power of prayer. Look for Christ. Look for Him so that His presence may permeate your body, your spirit, your soul. Just as the Jewish people who recorded in the Old Testament having had God's special presence overshadowing them throughout the forty years of Exodus, so will you, too, experience that cloud of God's visible, majestic Presence—His Shechinah. (Ex. 13:21, 22; Nb. 12:5)

No man can be making much of his life who has not a very definite conception of what he is living for. And if we were to ask a dozen men what the end of their life is, we would be surprised to find out how few have formed even a very dim idea. God has spoken to us through time. He has asked us to pray to Him as a friend would speak to a friend. We cannot be silent in such company. And speaking to such a friend is not mere conversation. It has a higher name. It is communion. It is *prayer*.

The fervent prayer of a religious man is far more effectual than a striking, cerebral, cold, formulated prayer; nor is it just a descriptive figure of speech nicely woven into a well-phrased paragraph. Faith in God, to Whom we pray, is much more important than the wording of the prayer. True prayer must contain the identity of ourselves and not be sanctimoniously feigned, as incense burning nowhere in its vanishing flight. *It must be from the heart that experiences wounds —wounds of its own, wounds of another.* The wording of our prayer is of secondary importance. Indeed Jesus Himself once indicated that words are not even necessary for an acceptable prayer. Words, however, do render expression to that which dwells in our hearts. They become only tools for our language with God. But the important thing to remember is that we must pray with spirit. Jesus Himself has taught us how to pray in His spirit:

> "I pray for them;
> I am not praying for the world
> But for those you have given me,
> because they belong to you." (Jn. 17:9)

11

TO HEAL AND TO BUILD

PART I

"To heal and to build is a noble task. Dig deep and sow good seed. To heal and to build in support of something worthy is, I believe, a noble task."

LYNDON BAINES JOHNSON
April 1, 1968, speech to the National Association
of Broadcasters

Healing Prayer

"Lord Jesus, as I kneel in prayer before Your Eucharistic Presence during the early hours of this morn I pray that You will take my mind with all its faculties and use them appropriately and influencingly concerning the thoughts that You would have me write. Lord, the world in which I live and to which I am exposed is a world of many wounds. Lord, You have called me to a healing apostolate that I may serve Your peoples through Your holy Church. Help me and all others who are called in like fashion to heal and to build.

Let the healing ministry, Lord, seek to rid the world of ignorance, ill health, personality disorders. We must, with God's grace, rid ourselves of this bitter inheritance. Lord, give me love and loyalty to the Church. Let me add to its increase: never to destroy or tarnish its life. Help me, Lord, to heal, not to injure; to help, not to hurt; to strengthen and sustain with patience, compassion, and trust."

Healing Through the Person of Jesus

"One day the apostles Peter and John, disciples of Jesus, were going to the Temple to pray. They passed a lame man begging for alms at the Temple gate. When the lame man asked alms of them, they focused their eyes intently upon him and said: 'Look at us!' "

One can almost sense with forceful sensitivity the expectancy of renewed hope rising within the heart and mind of this beggar. Though he was expecting to receive some monetary assistance from Peter and John, yet, nevertheless, the voices of the apostles who said: "Look at us!" seemed to stir a far greater expectancy. It was a feeling quite different. A stirring within the beggar's heart portended something extraordinary. But remembering the reality of his lameness, he merely stretched out his hand for some silver or gold. Peter addressed him further with all-the-more-promising emphasis: ". . . but Peter said, 'I have neither silver nor gold, but I will give you what I have: in the name of Jesus Christ the Nazarene, walk!' . . . and he went with them into the Temple, walking and jumping and praising God." (Ac. 3:6–8) What did Peter and John have? They had the person of Jesus living within them, and they gave Jesus to that man. And this is what every healing ministry that is divine must convey: the person of Jesus. There is power in the person of Jesus. Healing comes through the person and name of Jesus. "O Lord, may we never misuse Your healing gifts, but always find in them the true source of life and salvation: You, the healing love."

The Christian faith pivots on a person: Jesus Christ. If Jesus Christ is fully God and fully man, as He claimed to be, then to this Jesus Christ of Nazareth all human history is subject. As the Son of God, He claimed to be Our Lord; as the Son of Man, He claimed to be our model. And as fully God and fully man, He claimed to be our Redeemer. Many people came to Jesus during His public lifetime. The gospel tells of only a few: There was a centurion who sought help for a servant. A woman cried to be healed from the palsy. A man born blind wanted a miracle to see the created beauty of God. A boy was freed from his possession. A time-serving senator walked in the darkness of the night and left the presence of Jesus in the early-morning hours illumined by the light of a new birth. A man called Jairus obtained a new breath of life for his dying daughter. Old and young, the infirm, the powerful, the troubled, the influential, sinful, devout, poor, wealthy, the Jew, the Greek, pagans, every possible type representing the human status and condition came to Him, Who had authority over all creation.

The earthly ministry of Jesus Christ expressed itself precisely through three phases. Matthew 9:35 scripturally preserves for us Jesus' threefold ministry; Jesus went about teaching and preaching and healing. What this is saying is that, according to Matthew, specifically 4:23, Jesus went about all Galilee, teaching in the synagogues and preaching the gospel of the kingdom, and healing all manner of sickness among the people. When Christ blessed the sands of Palestine with His presence, none who witnessed Him attempted to deny His healing power. They may have questioned His authority to forgive sins.

Jesus, Source of Healing

The source of divine healing is Jesus Christ Himself. He Himself says: "I am the Way, the Truth and the Life." (Jn. 14:6) "I have come so that they may have life." (Jn. 10:10) Peter calls Him "the prince of life." (Ac. 3:15)

The healing love of the Father proceeds from the fullness of the Trinity's love for man. It descends through the person of Jesus Christ, Son of the Father and Redeemer of man, by the agency of the Holy Spirit, Third Person of the Blessed Trinity. Man, through a condition of faith, be it implicit or explicit, becomes receptive to the agency of healing, the Holy Spirit, Sanctifier of wounded seekers. One therefore can easily perceive that the healing ministry of prayer is truly Trinitarian: Father, Son, and Spirit, dwelling within the Christian.

Throughout the healing processes—although the Trinity is the major agent of healing love—man remains with his free will to accept or reject the healing love. Jesus Himself uttered: "Until now you have not asked for anything in my name. Ask and you will receive, and so your joy will be complete." (Jn. 16:24) The fullness of this joy in asking with faith is experienced through a variety of remarkable and marvelous healings. And what is more notably remarkable is that in no way does divine healing confine itself to physical illnesses: Its Trinitarian power tangibly penetrates every aspect of human life. Ultimately the most outstanding experience of healing focuses itself on the excitement and the joy of what it means to be a Christian. Christ Himself, through divine healing, reveals Himself with impelling impact as truly alive today. Through Him a man in search of healing undergoes a voyage of discovery through "inscape". In Christ the human soul is confronted with the meaning of one's life—his purpose for being. The ministry of healing, through its own unique power, tends to open a human searching heart to the love of the Trinity. The Trinity startles man with tremendous awareness of God Himself and of His love, which is Himself. In such an experience, the individual is presented with divine grace to overpower and conquer the apparent meaninglessness of life as well as the excruciating search for self-identity.

In the healing ministry, it is of paramount importance that one seek God for Himself and not just for His healing gifts. Hope and faith in God enable one to continue on in an unshakable conviction of God's will and power to heal. Herein lies one's best hope, even for physical healing. It is His grace in our lives that continuously sustains and empowers. God in His mercy offers for each one of us that special moment of healing through which a complete relinquishment of ourselves to Him becomes the true work of a miracle.

A foible of human nature is that those in dire need may seek balm for their wounds and forget Him who places the balm on their wounds. There is a danger that man may look for the healing without the Healer, and this would be contrary to divine healing. By way of simple example, suppose you visited a person and respected his gift more than him? What an insult! In such a case, there remains only an inverted value. With conscious responsibility to what God has made me and called me to, I would now recommend to you the direct object of your reading, your reflection, your assimilation, your search for means and techniques to apply to your own healing ministries: the *person of Jesus*.

1. Jesus is omniscient, that is, all-knowing. He never makes a mistake in His diagnosis.
2. Jesus is omnipresent. No matter where you are, He is at hand, ready, available.
3. Jesus is omnipotent, that is, all-powerful. There is nothing He cannot do.
4. Jesus is available to all, that is, He will not turn down a new client. He invites your trust.

In discussing the healing ministry, one cannot find enough repetition, even to the point of verbosity and the surrender of simple, direct style, to accent that a healing ministry is in no way an attempt to coerce an unwilling God to heal. Because of the versatility and variety of man's attitudes and dispositions, as well as personal intentions, it is necessary to reemphasize that the perfect will of God for wholeness must be fulfilled in us. God alone is the beginning of healing, and God alone is the ultimate end of healing. The Trinity offers Its healing blessings because of unbounded mercy and love. A human being cannot force God to heal. Just as God Himself cannot be forced, so He respects us by not coercing us. Nor will we coerce Him if true respect for the Godhead dwells within our soul. One of God's great revelations about His nature is that He heals out of pure compassion.

A soul in search of blessing approaches the throne of God with the power of prayer. Moreover, one approaches the throne of God through His Church so that whatever gift may be granted to him is truly God's healing love producing a wholeness unto Him.

Why Did Jesus Heal?

Jesus had a divine purpose for rendering healing. Two thirds of His public ministry was spent in healing love. From His very nature there flowed forth infinite compassion. The Scriptures emphasize very often that He was moved by compassion and healed the sick. (Mt. 14:14) In Matthew 20:29–34, two blind men cried for the miracle of sight. They called out for mercy. Jesus stopped and asked, by way of purifying their intentions, what they wanted. Was it alms or healing? Jesus had compassion on them and made them see the beauties of His Father's created world. What zealous passion Jesus had to do good! The very word passion itself carries the idea of suffering. The Latin verb *compatior* means "I suffer with." To feel the sorrow of another is very important. Do you remember the widow's son as Luke 7:11–15 depicts? Jesus had compassion on her. "Weep not," He consoled. How wonderful to know that our High Priest, Jesus, is in touch with our infirmities, as Paul so well reminds us. (Heb. 4:15)

Physical healing played a very important part in the ministry of Our Lord Jesus Christ. Outside of the Gospels, it would be very difficult to estimate what percentage of His time was spent in ministering to the sick. John 6:2 states: ". . . and a large crowd followed him, impressed by the signs he gave by curing the sick." From the very onset of His ministry there is recorded that Our Lord proclaimed that He came "to heal the broken-hearted, to preach deliverance to the captives, and recovery of sight to the blind." (Lk. 4:18) He also proclaimed Himself the Good Shepherd, that He had come that they might have life and that they might have it abundantly. He emphasized over and over again that He was the Good Shepherd and that the Good Shepherd surrenders His life for His sheep. He clearly illustrated that any shepherd who dares to be a shepherd must be a good manager, bearing in his mind one great objective: that his flock flourish. He also confirmed His person and His apostolate when He said that it was the Holy Spirit that had anointed Him. Peter himself reaffirmed this reality through his own preaching at Cornelius' house: "God had anointed him with the Holy Spirit and with power, and because God was with him, Jesus went about doing good and curing all who had fallen into the power of the devil." (Ac. 10:38) And so the healing love of Jesus for the sick was a definite part of His ministry. He healed through the power of the Holy Spirit.

Jesus also healed to fulfill prophecies. Hoping that it might be fulfilled, the prophet Isaiah had spoken: "He took our sicknesses away and carried our diseases for us." (Mt. 8:17) Jesus healed to prove that God had sent Him, for as Peter proclaimed on Pentecost Day, it was Jesus of Nazareth who had been approved by God

among them by the working of miracles, portents, and signs, which
God did by Him. (Ac. 2:22) Jesus also healed in order to enable the
healed to witness and to minister, not only to Christ Himself but to
the members of His body, the Church. And furthermore, Jesus
healed by imparting abundant life and, in so doing, destroying the
influence of Satan. Whatever the reasons may be, all of them
proclaimed the ultimate purpose of divine healing: to manifest the
works of God. This last reason is the most important of all: the
glory of God. The chief end of man is to glorify God. Each one of
us should seek things that glorify our Father in heaven. We should
unite ourselves to those things and elements, those persons and
events of life, that show how wonderful God really is.

Jesus chose apostles and other disciples to continue His work. He
taught them how to use His healing power of love when He said,
". . . they will lay their hands on the sick, who will recover." (Mk.
16:18)

God the Father loves us. We are His children. God the Father
sent His Son, Jesus Christ, to proclaim the Good News. The compassionate love of Jesus is proclaimed in His Word: to open the eyes
of the blind, to give hearing to the deaf and speech to the dumb,
and to set captives free. (Lk. 4:18) Because of His compassionate
love, Jesus heals.

The Church as Healer

One concept of Christian healing is related to the charism of
evangelization. The Christian message of salvation presents sickness
as connected with original sin (see Jn. 9:2–3), rather than personal sin. Scriptural history factually narrates that the first man and
woman of the human race had been victimized by the deceptive
forces of Satan. After that fall into a state of original sin, the prog-
eny that followed was itself, by transmission of human life, sub-
jected to the state of the original wound. For this reason all humanity on earth experience the sufferings consequent upon sin.

The original sin is an enemy of humanity, from conception onward. We dwell on the planet earth with a depersonalized, fallen,
and weakened human nature. Since, therefore, the original state of
sinfulness produces a spiritual sickness, there arises in contrast the

healing cure that must itself be spiritual. This spiritual antidote to the spiritual infirmity of man is ministered by Christ, the Divine Physician, through His Church.

Original sin has not only affected us on a general basis but has also affected each human being through specific personal transgressions. Each soul has its own story to narrate. Within the pages of one's own autobiography are written a host of human infractions with specific causative factors. Again, an antidote offering remedy becomes personal. During His earthly ministry of healing, Our Blessed Lord ministered to individuals of every conceivable background. As each one approached the Divine Physician with his individual and personal need, Jesus applied the appropriate method.

In whatever way healing is applied, the common ingredient in remedy is prayer. Christ promised to apply His healing balm to all men for all times. The channel of His healing administration, most elite in its origin, is His bride, the Church. Jesus had many ways of applying His healing. At times there was the utilization of the *laying on of hands*. He offered this sacramental healing rite to His Church. "They shall lay hands on the sick and they shall recover." (Mk. 16:18)

As imposing as the laying on of hands may be, and Jesus used this method (Lk. 4:40), He never enslaved Himself to it as the only means to heal. The Scriptures narrate a multiplicity of ways. Each situation and each personality warranted its own treatment. At other times the Master was seen to cure the sick simply by His *touch*. The story of the widow of Naim's son bears such compassion and tenderness. (Lk. 7:11–15) Again Jesus is seen as drawing the best from the Canaanite woman's daughter. (Mt. 15:21–28) The power that was used therein was the tremendous force of *intercessory prayer*. At still other times, the Scriptures depict the Divine Physician as going about His healing mission by *anointing*, as in the case of the blind man. (Jn. 9:6–7) Above and beyond the multiple ways of curing the sick that Jesus used, there stands out prominently the most beautiful of all: healing through the *forgiveness of sins*, healing by *exorcism*. Both means, tremendous in power as they are emphatically dramatized by the scriptural writers, describe acutely and pointedly the essential value of the healing ministry.

One therefore can perceive that particular illnesses, particular temperaments, must be treated appropriately. At times, it is the sacramental healing rites that are utilized. At other times, the strength producing cures flows from private or communal prayer, by petition and intercession. I have been told that God has even utilized unorthodox methods for healing. Some of these methods serve solely as points of contact. Some of these are radio, television, telephone, or prayer-line telephone ministries, and other religiously oriented media. Another tremendous tool used quite extensively in our contemporary age for evangelism and the continuation of gospel blessings is that of the cassette ministry. There are no limitations to God's infinite love for man as His spirit enraptures the world of His best creation, bringing about the healing of man.

The Church offers many splendid rites in its healing administration. The most splendid, in my opinion, is that of the sacrament of the Holy Eucharist. I have witnessed in many of my services innumerable healings through this sacrament. Both on the local scene and in the outreach ministry, whenever feasible and prudent, my ministry of healing is conducted in the presence of the Holy Eucharist. The power of the Word, the power of healing, cannot be felt more impressively than when huge multitudes from all walks of life bask in the rays of the Eucharistic Christ. Hearts are warmed, minds are prayerfully reflective, love emanates from hearts that have forgotten how to love, forgiveness flows forth as each particular soul, individual as it may be amid a throng of thousands of participants, remains in awe before Him Who is called the Eucharistic King and Prisoner of Love.

The Church of Christ offers other forms of consolation and compassion as it seeks to heal the wounds of its children. Adjacent to the life of its sacraments, there are the Church's own institutions of sacramentals. Christians, besides seeking recovery from illnesses by means of medical care, have always believed in the efficacy of prayer and religious blessings through secondary sacramental rites. It is interesting to peruse the book of the Roman Catholic Ritual. Therein one finds countless blessings. There are sensitive prayers in behalf of the sick and the dying, for children and adults in hospitals and nursing homes, and many others. The Christian tradition is rich with its language of prayer. The Church has always voiced its cries to God, beseeching His divine touch upon the human condition.

Religious anthropology has supported the fact that both non-Christians and Christians have always sought cures for sickness through some form of sacrifice or even of libation. The Old Testament is replete with such examples. For instance, pagans would deem it necessary to pour out onto the ground precious oil or water or some other valued liquid. This would be done in a spirit of jubilation and thanksgiving for conquests made. As these offerings were presented, a spirit of sacrifice was rendered to the gods of their knowledge, such as to the sun, the moon, the goddess of fire, the goddess of love. Anthropological studies also reveal the prevalence of human sacrifice among the pagans. Often it is read that vestal virgins were taken from an early age, preserved, nurtured, and educated until the proper moment of sacrifice presented itself. These oblations of human life, according to the human understanding, served as oblations of thanksgiving, adoration, reparation, and petition.

In severing ourselves from pagan practices, we see that religious persons are prone to seek out trustworthy people who may intercede with God for them. People have an inner urge to identify themselves and their needs with such people of prayer. So often we see countless persons turn to a priest, minister, or rabbi with the beautiful and touching plea "Please pray for me!" What a sense of responsibility rests upon each one of us who has distinctively been called to the life of intercessory prayer!

To whom else are these people to turn? In the Old Testament, one turned to the prophets, who were intercessors between the person and God. The sick would be seen coming for healing prayer, for healing touch from those persons who appeared as specifically blessed to deal with the respective needs of the people. The Scriptures are replete with stories of sick persons seeking out the prophets, who in turn would implore healing as a grace upon life. Miraculous cures are recorded everywhere in the Old Testament. For example, in the Second Book of Kings there is the story of the widow whose son was called back to life by Elisha the prophet. (2 K. 4-5) There is also the healing of Naaman from leprosy, along with the concept that sickness is often attributed to the devil.

Such an idea was prevalent in those times. On the other hand, in the New Testament, Jesus fulfills the presence of the Father and restores the laws of God. Christ appears as person and as power. Christ's miraculous healing of the sick is one of the signs that the last, Messianic times are coming, according to Matthew 11:4-5. In other words, what is meant is that there can be no other New Testament. The New Testament is Jesus Christ, Son of God, fulfilling His purpose. Not only He Himself but also His chosen apostles were selected to heal the sick. (Mt. 10:1)

The charism of healing manifests itself in miraculous cures brought about by the apostles as recorded, for example, in Acts 3:1–8. (cf. also James 5:14–16) The presbyters anointed the sick not only for bodily cures but also for spiritual regeneration. The Church later recognized the anointing of the sick as a sacrament. Yet this was already happening when the apostles went out, laying on hands and anointing as they said, "Rise and be healed." In the early Church, St. James's text was invoked to justify the liturgical anointing of the sick by bishops or priests, for spiritual and bodily healings —and that is the sacrament—as well as private anointings by sick persons themselves and others, mainly for recovery. In the early Church there were not enough priests or bishops to go around anointing, so people used to have little bottles of oil which the priests had blessed. These oils would be brought home and kept between candles or in a little sanctuary. The father or the mother would take this oil and bless the family with it. There was implicit belief that some healing takes place through prayer. If we visit the catacombs, we see the pictures and writings on the walls that tell us that the people of that time thought that their prayers meant something. These first prayers depicted in the art of the catacombs serve to teach us a great deal about theology.

For too long, the healings and other miracles of Jesus have been used in an apologetic way, seeking to prove that He was divine. Even though Jesus did appeal to His works as a sign of His authenticity, He was always reticent about His power to heal. He continually identified His work as a direct object to communicate the fullness of His Father's loving His children by sending the presence of His Son to mankind. It was the whole person, body, soul and spirit that came to Jesus in his or her broken humanity. It was the broken, wounded seeker in all of his and her forms of illness and disease that cried out and spoke most beseechingly to the merciful Jesus. Jesus touched them as Yahweh, for, as His name, Jesus, indicates, He was the One Who saves. It was God, through Jesus Christ, Who wanted all of us to enjoy, as total beings, total health both within ourselves and through our relationships. All that Jesus required from those who came to Him was the condition of believing in His love and His power to heal sick persons. The second element that Jesus insisted upon was that element which every apostolate of prayer for healing must have: the propagation of the faith and the "propaganda of the faith." Herein lies conversion. Jesus insisted that the deep faith in His power to heal all sicknesses is really the turning of one's life over completely to His dominion as Jesus Christ and Lord.

Jesus instructs those who believe in Him: "Go and heal." He empowered His followers to go forth and teach and bring to others His own healing power that He gave them. He promised such power to them that they would do even greater things, because He and His Father would abide with the Holy Spirit. (Jn. 14:25–26) The true followers of Jesus down through the ages have, therefore, accepted in faith His commission to go forth. In His saving name, that powerful name of Jesus, they went forth; they taught and they prayed. The results, the effects, the manifestations were healings and other miracles that became stepping-stones for evangelization. And as in the first century, by these acts of power, people have received the gift of faith through conversion. The baptized members of the Church, both the hierarchy and the laity, believe that Jesus continues His healing ministry and that He has passed on a tremendously special responsibility to preach the Word and to heal the sick.

A sad outcome of the apparent lethargy of healing prayer occurred when Emperor Constantine accepted Christianity as the official religion of the Roman Empire. When suffering, such as martyrdom and persecution, was somewhat diminished, the people became complacent, and Christians began to pray less for healing. Monasteries, a faulty Platonism, and other puritanical forces entered and influenced the minds with false ascetics. A misconstrued theology of illness was introduced as redemptive suffering. There was also a diminution of praying for healing as the sacrament for the anointing of the sick was introduced and evolved. But God, Who has the welfare of His people always at hand, has waited out the time He granted us and has restored to us in our contemporary age the practice of the early Church of praying for the sick and seeing healing as applicable to the total person.

And so today we know the experience of compassion, peace, and restoration not only for those who are at the point of death but also for those who may fall ill, as well as those who need the forgiveness of sin. And by emphasizing the healing of all sicknesses, the Church manifests its external care for the sick as it sends forth its priests to witness the power of Jesus' commission. (*See* Mk. 16:18) On other occasions, priests and laity are overjoyed that Christ is alive through them as they lay hands on the members of their families, relatives, and friends and even at times use blessed oil, *not that of the sacrament*, while rejoicing that the sick who come to them or whom they may visit are restored as total persons.

Through His gift of healing to His Church, Christ offers to all mankind His healing love. The Church is very conscious of its healing love through those channels of grace which make us like unto Christ. These are the seven rivers of blood that flow as sacramental life from the wounded side of Christ from whence the Church took its life. These are the sacraments of the Church: Baptism, Confirmation, Holy Eucharist, Reconciliation, the Anointing of the Sick, Marriage, and Priesthood.

The red rivers of redemptive blood that flow from the wounds of Jesus have been appropriately compared to the seven stages of man. By His passion, Christ has merited for all men the gift of grace. This gift of grace leads to salvation and to the eternal beatific vision. If man is to be saved, this grace must be applied to his being. Christ Himself applies God's grace to every man who seeks. Jesus does this through His Church. The Church, as Christ instituted it, is the continuation and extension of the Christ Himself throughout the ages of time. Christ has ascended into heaven. Nevertheless, He has promised to be with us realistically. And through His Church, He continues to distribute and shower grace to all men. His Church is His bride; His Church is His Mystical Body. Jesus' love for men is infinite. Being prepared always to give grace from heaven to those who will sincerely repent, recognize Him, proclaim Him in faith and in love, He has instituted a visible channel of His life to man through the sacraments.

To repeat, Christ instituted seven sacraments: Baptism, Confirmation, the Holy Eucharist, Penance, Anointing of the Sick, Holy Orders, and Matrimony. I emphasize this so that, being impressed by their number, we may understand their individual application to the differing needs of the seven stages of man. We can see that they show a parallel between the life of grace and the natural life of man.

St. Thomas, if I may simplify, in his *Summa*, states that before a man can live at all, he must be born. But before he can live spiritually in Christ he must also be born in the life of grace. Baptism offers this spiritual birth. Secondly, St. Thomas states that man must grow to maturity so that he can do a man's work. In terms of the spiritual order, this growth is necessary, and so the sacrament of Confirmation confers this strength that aids man in his spiritual combat against the forces of self-destruction and depersonalization. Just as physical man survives with nourishment so as to preserve life and to obtain strength, so the Holy Eucharist—containing the true body and blood of Jesus—serves as a sacrament in the spiritual order. Life objectively demonstrates that all men become victims of illness and disease. As they search to be cured and restored to their former vitality, through the use of natural means, so in the spiritual sphere man becomes ill through personal and social sins. Jesus offers restoration to spiritual health through the consoling sacrament of Penance, wherein sin is realistically and objectively forgiven by God Himself. As man inevitably must die, he comes to the judgment seat of God with the remains of sin, unless he has done adequate penance on earth for his responsible and deliberate violations. Through the sacrament of the Anointing of the Sick, a man is restored to spiritual vigor, the remains of sin are cleansed away, and he is prepared for the eternal embrace of a welcoming Christ. Since he is a social being, man needs leadership to oversee the dealings and the public acts of the community. Apropos of the Church, God's people, the sacrament of Holy Orders offers a hierarchical leadership whereby priests offer sacrifices and prayer and distribute the sacramental life of Jesus. The most common vehicle by which men travel the earth is the sacred bond and unity of the marriage vocation. God blessed marriage, that it would propagate the human race. Arduous indeed are the paths of the marriage vocation, wherein personalities completely different seek their own sanctification and salvation as well as the prosperity of their family life before God and man. In order to assist this holy marriage contract, Jesus blesses the obligations and the accomplishments of the marriage state of holy espousals.

A sacrament, as the name implies, "is an outward sign instituted by Christ to give grace." The sacraments receive their power to give grace from God through the merits of Jesus Christ, Who died and atoned for us on the cross. All the sacraments give sanctifying grace.

And each of the seven sacraments gives a special, individual grace. This is called sacramental grace.

A sacrament dramatizes God's sanctification of man/woman. Its effects are twofold: a consecration/a making of man/woman a member of Christ and rendering this Christian soul into a sacred minister in the Church or a special union with the Church. Though, generally speaking, sacramental grace produces sanctifying life (grace) in each soul, as well as the virtues, the gifts of the Holy Spirit, and actual grace, *each sacrament gives a special grace appertaining to the specific individual sacrament administered.* For example, according to the teachings of St. Thomas Aquinas on the sacraments, baptism is directed to the spiritual rebirth of a man and his incorporation in the Church as a member of the body of Christ.

Sacramental grace is special: In theological schools of discernment, it is believed that sacramental grace gives permanent powers as a remedy for the weaknesses produced in man by sin. Other circles of theological thought believe that sacramental grace gives a special feature of actual graces which are necessary for man to attain *the distinct holiness for which each sacrament is directed.* The sacraments always give grace to him who receives them with the right disposition.

The seven sacraments are the channels of Christ's grace for mankind. *The graces of these sacraments heal the wounds and sicknesses of one's soul, make it more beautiful and pleasing to God, and even give new and eternal life.* As we reflect over the days of our lives, as we remember the many times the Church has blessed us, may we look up to heaven and thank Our Lord, Jesus, for having given us on Calvary's heights those precious red rivers of His grace: His channels of life, purchased by the anguish of crucifixion.

The sacrament of the sick was formally recognized in the eleventh and twelfth centuries (several things were promulgated in that period, including the law of celibacy), when the doctrine of the sacraments became explicit in the awareness of the Church. The anointing of the sick as a sacrament was counted among the seven ecclesiastic sacraments, and bodily healing came to be considered as a subordinate and conditional effect. In order to understand the gifts of healing, we need only to go back to the sacrament of the sick in the eleventh century and ask ourselves what was done before the eleventh century for healing. Charism! The charism of healing is rec-

ognized in the Church whenever miraculous cures are effected by
people whom God calls. Like myself, you don't have to be holy for
God to work through you. It would help, but God is going to bring
about His gift regardless of the person. The sacrament works by itself, whether the person is in the state of grace or not. But woe to
that person who dares to minister the works of the Lord without
Him, who does God's work fraudulently—*Maledictus qui fecit opus
Domini fraudulenter*.

No sacrament has been more feared or neglected than the one
which was known as Extreme Unction, or with its more frightening
designation, Last Rites. Countless Catholics did not have the opportunity to witness this rite; and because it seemed to be surrounded
by confessional secrecy, increased trepidation permeated the Catholic mind. The phrase Extreme Unction was introduced in the
twelfth century. When it was applied, it took the stance that an
anointed person was at the point of death or in the danger of death
and that such a person would not recover from sickness. In fact, the
canonical injunction was that the danger of death had to be a prerequisite for the administration and reception of this sacrament. It
takes time to erase misunderstandings; and the new rite, for an opportunity of restoration to health, is now called the Anointing of the
Sick. The Vatican Council was pleased to offer to its children the
new, revised rite, approved in 1972 and effected in 1974. In so doing,
the Council hoped to transmit the beauty and dynamics of such a
powerful sacrament and rid it of its lingering smell of death.

Thus, healing has emerged as an important part of Church life
and as a definite power contained in Christianity. In the renewed liturgy of the sacraments of the Church, the sacrament of the Anointing of the Sick has been now rendered to accent more appropriately
the essence and the nature of this anointing: It stresses its healing
power.

As I have pointed out before, there has always been a deep belief
in the Catholic Church in the power of prayer for obtaining
healings. Prayers have been written and proclaimed both privately
and publicly for seeking cures on the physical, the psychic, and the
spiritual levels. The Church seeks substantial healing. Man's psychological problem is man's separation from himself. This separation
affects his thoughts, his self-image, and his relationship with the

world. Man, as a person, enjoys the faculties and operations of thinking, acting, and feeling. Each person is a unit. It is the duty of those called to heal to seek to bring into harmony and oneness all these parts—not as a sum total, but as a display of balance, integration, and unity.

The Church, even though it places its accent on the spiritual, cannot ignore the other integral elements of man. In its healing ministry, the Church with full knowledge of its power constantly emphasizes the totality of man in his need for healing. The Church in its many apostolates attunes itself to the various facets or aspects of the soul (body, mind, and spirit). Those who deal with the body, mind, and spirit recognize the interdependency of one to another. They also detect that illness in any one of these areas affects the other parts. For example, the mind can create pain in one's stomach; an ulcer in the stomach can upset the emotion of pleasure and bring dejection to the mind. People should be made aware of the totality of their being. They should recognize the unity of their physical and emotional constitution. Those rendering service in the healing professions are increasingly developing and maturing their outlook in terms of the whole person. Extensive research and experience are confirming this new outlook regarding the interrelationship of body, mind and spirit. If healing be truly authentic, it must refer to the whole person. And although healing of the body is important, it is not all-important. Its healing certainly is of worth, but not of supreme worth. Those blessed with the gift of healing focus all their energies not only on the body and the psyche, but ultimately on the soul.

As Christ accented the healing of the person, so the Church, in the footsteps of Christ, stresses the same substantial healing. True spirituality which is the substantial healing in the Church has a relationship both to God and to our separation from our fellow men. The Church, in its true concept of *ecclesia*, reflects its functioning as that which is "called out" of a lost humanity. As each generation unfolds itself in social, psychological, and economic realms, man himself is recognizing that he as man is less than he knows he should be. Today's generation recognizes this. Nevertheless the problem is not new; ever since the fall of rebellious man, *rebellious man* has been and has acted that way. And the Church, therefore, is called out of this humanity to be a regenerated humanity before a lost humanity. Though physically the body of Jesus rose from the dead on Easter, yet the body of Christ found its birth on Pentecost. "Just as a human body, though it is made up of many parts, is a single unit because all these parts, though many, make one body, so it is with Christ. In the one Spirit we were all baptized, Jews as well as Greeks, slaves as well as citizens, and one Spirit was given to us all to drink." (1 Co. 12:12–13) And so, therefore, with the Pentecost birth, the body of Christ was born in a particular form. It is in a very specific way His body.

Being His body, the Church is called out to exhibit Him to the world, until He returns. Just as our own human bodies are our means of communication to the external world, so the Church as the body of Christ should be Christ's means of communication to the external world. When we speak and act our interior thoughts through our bodies, they become our point of communication with the external world. Through such a medium we thus affect the world. The Church, as the physical body of Christ, is called to be the means whereby He, Christ, may be exhibited. The Church is Christ's means, by which He acts, performs, heals, renews, builds afresh the external world, until He comes again. The Church should be the reality of Christ and the exhibition of His presence to each generation.

Christ is alive in His Church with His presence by the charisms. The charisms are for each generation. There have never been nor will there ever be, until the end of time, a generation without charisms, because His presence will never be denied through these vital and personifying manifestations. Each one of us, therefore, must look into our hearts and consciences.

The external witnessing of Christ to His Church requires a substantial restored relationship between men. This restored relationship exists not only between God and man through spiritual healing, not only between the individual and himself as in psychological healing (and this is quite crucial), but between man and man as socially related to the Christian community. This process is the vocation and apostolate of authentic and valid healing existing in the Church of Christ.

God's spirit of concern will always hover over His Church through all ages. The Church is Christ's true love. It is His people. He seeks that oneness of wholeness and holiness. When Jesus was on earth, He spent all His time doing good for people. He went about doing good, and healing all that were oppressed of the devil. (see Ac. 10:38) He loved people and was always interested in healing them. Nothing was too insignificant for Him to be concerned about. He was always where the people were hurting. He has not changed. "Jesus Christ is the same today as he was yesterday and as he will be for ever." (Heb. 13:8) He is concerned about all of us, you and me, here and now. He really sees and cares for us with watchful concern. Just give Him that chance, and you will see His power drive away everything and anything that depersonalizes you.

And so God is with us through His Church, through His Christ, Who dwells in it, always alive! The Church, with Christ, therefore is replete with gifts of all sorts, because the Church has THE CHRIST, WHO IS THE GIFT. God knows the distinctive needs proper to our time. Some sects are intent today on speaking of the Church as near to the end. However, whether the Book of the Apocalypse—or the Book of Revelation, as it is also called—be relevant to this age or not, the fact remains that the Church in general (exclusive of no religious Christian sect) is now enjoying her healing apostolate with ever more joy. Perhaps with the Book of Revelation and its contents in focus, these manifestations of healing may be expressive of an age that is in deep need of evangelization. Moreover, the Church today is recognizing and appropriating with greater enthusiasm this gift of healing as an integral part of the total gospel for wholeness. Some of these blessings of healing activate instantaneous cures; others, a gradual or progressive recovery.

The Church of Christ lives from the wounded side of Jesus, Who, dying on the cross, gave to the world the birth of renewal. From that sacred side pierced by the love of man that had turned into hatred, came forth the living sacraments of God's most precious treasure. We are cleansed in His blood. Ephesians 5:25–27 tells us: "Christ loved the Church and gave Himself up for her to make her holy, purifying her in the bath by the power of the Word, to present to Himself a glorious Church, holy and immaculate, without stain or wrinkle or anything of that sort."

As we kneel at the foot of the crucifix, as we try to pray as a means to capture the throbbing heartbeat of a God come to earth and put to death for no other crime except an excessive amount of love, we cannot help but proclaim:

> Jesus, Your sacred heart was pierced with a lance,
> And from it poured forth blood and water that Your
> Church might come forth into birth.
>
> R.D.O.

As we continue to kneel at the foot of the crucifix and look up into the dying eyes of Christ, we cannot find words to express adequately the gratitude within our hearts.

The Spirit of the Apostolate of Prayer for Healing

Having established the person of Jesus as the source of healing, I now feel comfortable in presenting the following reflections in reference to the healing apostolate. And so within Part II of this chapter I will relate the foregoing thoughts to some of the powerful strengths, insights, and dynamics that God has transferred to His people in the utilization of the Apostolate of Prayer for Healing, of which I am Director.

During the past year or so, some bishops, many priests, religious men and women, numerous doctors, and other colleagues medically inclined have asked me continually to write about these inner sources that are the underlying power and strength in my ministry of healing and evangelization. Such a project is quite arduous and far vaster than can be accomplished in one chapter or even one book. However, the responsibility to disseminate what God has done to me warrants public expression of the inner dynamics working both consciously and subconsciously within the gift beneath the man graced by God. In justice, therefore, to those who sincerely and with honest effort treat the countless sicknesses of humanity, I hope with all my heart to share that spirit of healing with which God has authentically blessed my once insignificant life. His grace alone uses me in the present position that He has allowed. It is, therefore, my one desire—and I cannot say this often enough—that God's glory and honor be praised by those who read, and that the Church to which I am espoused by dedication and priestly consecration be enriched and esteemed. It is also my purposeful intent to convey comprehensive and authentic knowledge concerning the spirit of health to my brother priests, to professional men dedicated to the field of medicine, and to all those of the laity who seek to alleviate the wounds of mankind that are deep and fundamental.

The purpose of divine healing is not only to offer compassionate love to an individual. The ultimate purpose of the healing must be theological, not medical. As in the case with the paralytic, for example (Lk. 5:18–26), there clearly was the proof of what God was doing to this paralytic's soul by helping his broken body. Like other incidents in both the Old Testament and the New Testament, many healing blessings were performed before the people through dramatic means. Today's scrutinizing eye as well as today's contemporary terminology might critically label healing signs of all sorts as "sensationalism." But whatever one wishes to call them, they nevertheless remain in fact and in truth an opportunity, a grace externally enacted with the precise intention *to teach a twofold lesson.* Healing-ministry circles would recognize and identify such double lessons as:

One—to authenticate the person being used to perform the healings.

Two—to illustrate the Word for renewal.

God works His mysteries of charism through us as one would blow air through a flute to produce a melody. Our motto for the Apostolate of Prayer for Healing is *Sanatio hominis . . . propaganda fidei;* i.e., the external manifestation of healing serving as a stepping-stone for the teaching and evangelizing of the faith.

The Spirit of Medicine and Healing

The medical profession looks upon the spirit of health as a restorative power of nature. It looks upon it as an energy always at hand, awaiting only an opportunity to enter in to make whole, and to harmonize all discords in the body. The psychologist, along with the religiously oriented, go beyond the body and look into the soul,

with its emotions, interpersonal relationships, and spiritual relationships of faith, hope, and love of God as well as of man. In a
united whole, therefore, we come upon holistic healing.

While the concept of holistic health is relatively new to the
health-care system, the idea of "holism" and its implications for our
human condition have been influential for thousands of years.
Holism refers to the theory that whole entities such as human
beings have an existence and a reality greater than the sum of their
parts. Applying the term holistic to the concept of health means
that achieving and maintaining good health involves much more
than just taking care of all the various components that make up the
physical body. For, as just stated, an individual is much more than
just the sum of his individual parts. In my perception and thinking,
such a unity is similar to an osmosis. I perceive it as an integration
of the physical, the mental, and the spiritual. All together, therefore,
they are in unison to form a unique being. And so what we can conclude in the concept of holistic health is that one can experience a
sense of well-being when there is a proper balance and understanding of body, mind, and spirit. If a person, moreover, is a
totality, not just a component of parts, then those who would offer
themselves as channels of healing realize that they must deal with a
total person. They must not deal with people just as areas that seem
to be out of balance. They must not deal with people merely as
symptoms or situations, for these manifest themselves only as abnor-
malities. These are intimately entwined as expressions with the person's whole being, and to such a degree that the function of all
levels is affected. Those who would deal with healing love should be
guided, encouraged, and directed to raise themselves as well as the
client's consciousness to spiritual reality, wherein all healing power
originates. In so doing, the ideal in holistic health produces itself as
the realization of a person's human potential, as a total being. It
offers such a person the profoundest desire to live a fulfilling and
satisfying life. It offers one not only the goal to be "well" in the
physical body but to be in harmony with oneself and with one's environment at all levels.

It is my hope that these meditations and reflections will not be
read merely by curiosity seekers or by the inquisitive erudite seeking
only a new technique for the furtherance and enhancement of their
own interest. It is this author's prayer, foremost and above all, that

the good and welfare of the broken body of Christ, members of the Church, be touched and blessed by all men and women who would sincerely offer to another human person the compassionate touch of healing love. Perhaps you will here find insights to be prayerfully studied, reflected, digested, and applied as you go forth to another's needs. If one approaches these chapters with responsible thought, then invigorating cognitive processes, new currents of mature understanding, will ensue for the healing of one's body, soul, and spirit. The result will be a spiritual digestion, an inner illumination, a holistic approach to healing. In so doing, the conduct of healer will seek to heal, not to injure; to help, not to hurt; to strengthen and sustain with patience, compassion, and trust.

The mercy of God's healing love can be applied anywhere in the world: in cities, towns, villages, homes, hospitals, leprosaria. God's mercy can be found on the back streets of ghettos, even in the back streets of Calcutta. I remember an editorial once that depicted very clearly an old temple in the back streets of Calcutta that was dedicated to the bloody goddess Kali. Next to the temple was a hospital. But it was a different kind of hospital. Outside, along its streets, there were people, part of the millions who live in the streets. They were poor and simple. But inside the hospital there was a different world. This hospital is a home for dying destitutes, and one of the persons who cares so much about these discarded ones is a Roman Catholic nun named Mother Teresa. If one were to visit and share in this corner of the world, one would see the nurses tenderly cleansing wounds, touching leprous stumps. It is quiet there. There is no crying. The eyes of many bedridden persons are not fearful. Those eyes belong to those who somehow, in spite of anguish, became secure and contented. The old people and the little children have a home there. They are wanted, and they are loved. One could not help but remember the words of Matthew 25:40: "And the King will answer, 'I tell you solemnly, in so far as you did this to one of the least of these brothers of mine, you did it to me.'"

The Problem of Pain

To be ill—to be really ill—frequently brings awareness, for the first time, of the frailties of the flesh and the limited span of human life. Pain is a signal of danger. The British author C. S. Lewis, in his book *The Problem of Pain*, says that pain announces ". . . something is wrong and needs diagnosis and healing." He also states: "God whispers to us in our pleasure, speaks in our conscience, and shouts in our pain." But, for most people, pain that racks one physically or mentally goes far beyond being a warning signal. For so many, it becomes a disease in itself. It can destroy the personality. Some pain can be alleviated. Some of it cannot. But all pain is sending us a message. In my own thinking, the pain of man that is touched by the Apostolate of Prayer for Healing offers him the message of evangelization: to be renewed in a refreshing baptism of the spirit toward a new behavior and activity that leads to sanctification and the crowning glory of eternal life.

The thoughtful Christian confronted with illness necessarily must wonder about the relationship of this affliction to his faith. He seeks an answer to what is the place of disease in this world that a supposedly good God created. He wonders at times, perhaps because of bad religious influence and misguidance, whether this illness may be a retribution from a stern and vindictive Creator. He questions his lack of faith, he tortures his mind over his innate sinfulness, he wonders whether his religious practices stand before God as defective. Consciously or subconsciously, both normal people and those seriously ill harbor such guilt feelings. But, to a doctor, be he Christian or not, sickness and disease as it manifests itself is a reality of a biological order. It is simply the body's way of responding to an injury.

With every pain that touches man, there must come to man a response to this tragedy. Although we as human persons grow into the maturity of facing life and even use the misfortune, only occasionally does the full reality of evil shock us into an awareness of wasted power and beauty and a thwarted destiny. Then we question shrilly, as did the second-century contemporaries of Tertullian: *Unde malum et quare?*—"Whence comes evil and why is it permitted?" St. Augustine's great contribution to philosophy was to point out that evil, though real, was not a real thing. As Aquinas put it: "Evil according as it is evil is not something in things, but is the privation of some particular good, inhering in some particular good." (*De Malo*, q. 1, as. 1) Evil is not a being but must exist in a being.

Chesterton says that we should love even that which is ugly, love that which is loveless.

Nevertheless, there remain anguish, disease, corruption, spiritual aridity, lack of peace of soul. And because it is pain, it is very essential to all evil. C. S. Lewis wrote: "Pain insists on being attended to." When one hurts, one seeks to have the hurt removed. Regardless of the pain we may suffer, there is no predicament that we cannot ennoble either by doing or by enduring. Christ is the response of healing to all pain. Christians, unlike the pagans, look to the cross of Jesus, bypass the cross to His resurrection power, see Him ascended unto heaven as Intercessor, and thereupon are nourished with a living faith that operates through a charity they have learned from the person of Jesus Christ their Lord. Through Jesus they learn how to avoid evil and how to conquer death.

Pain in search of healing calls for a physician. The word "physician" implies much the same as "doctor" in our English language. The healing word R A P H A, as seen in Exodus 15:26, ". . . for it is I, Yahweh, who give you healing," indicates the Divine Healer, Who is God. This name is given to reveal our redemptive privilege of being healed. This is not only a promise made by God, but it is *a statute and an ordinance.*

Healing as a Definition

Perhaps at this moment a proper definition of healing can now be construed. All things considered, one can state that healing contains a power from above that produces restoration to full health of one who is sick—be it in body or mind, spirit, and soul. The Apostolate of Prayer for Healing seeks DIVINE HEALING AND DIVINE RESTORATION OF MAN'S SPIRITUAL RELATIONSHIP TO HIS GOD, PSYCHOLOGICAL GROWTH TO MAN'S OWN PERSONAL SELF-ACCEPTANCE, HIS EMOTIONAL INTERPERSONAL RELATIONSHIP TO SOCIETY, AND RENEWED PHYSICAL VITALITY LOST BY DISEASE OR ACCIDENT. Through such an apostolate, one chosen by God becomes a vessel of God, according to the measure of God's outpouring gift, that allows healing and restoration to flow into the lives of thousands. (Cf. Ep. 4:11)

These definitions include restoration or recovery resulting from medical attention and spontaneous remission of some afflicting pain or disease. Healing also incorporates the power to improve a patient's bearing, outlook on his own status of being, or health, even if no physical amelioration is possible. Healing also affects a person positively by correcting the sick person's misconception about the very nature of his or her illness. In reference to psychic disorders, be they psychological disturbances or in the order of sociopathology, the term is applied to describe an improved or totally renewed mental status.

One of the areas of healing is that of deliverance. Although such a ministry is quite intriguing, it is nevertheless also dangerous. The essence of such a ministry pertains to the areas of obsessions or possessions (the latter being rare but nevertheless real). Those who are called to such an apostolate will realize that the causative factors are spiritual in nature, requiring spiritual means to be employed. In reference to healing as it is understood strictly in the medical sense, one is dealing with organic and functional facets. Identification of these is clearly perceived by examination and diagnosis. For appropriate treatment of such illnesses, this approach is necessary, because if we are to understand healing in its true and authentic role, then its primary medical connotation would be properly understood as to a restoration to normalcy in cases of organic illnesses.

As in the natural order of healing one must submit oneself to the processes of the medical profession, so, too, any conditions claiming "miraculous" healing must present themselves to the same scrutinizing discernment.

Again we repeat that the author of healing is God alone. "God alone is He Who heals all our diseases." (Ps. 103:3; Ac. 3:12–16) But even so, when medical attention is given and surgical skill is applied, still God remains as the ULTIMATE CAUSE OF THE HEALING. God, however, does use visible channels for His presence. He uses men and women, be they trained or untrained, to do His work. (Rm. 13:1–5) For the welfare of mankind, God requires such men and women to utilize "good and ethical means," either of the natural order or of the spiritual order. True Christian belief sees God as encouraging the use of good available means, whether they be medicine, surgery, chemotherapy, transfusions, and so forth, to prevent death and to prolong life. If God did not will our health until that moment in which He as Author of life calls us to the "big healing," eternity, then our Christian system of social agencies, hospitals, leprosaria, nursing homes, etc., would be a sham. These would only impose themselves as organizations laden with the burdens of monetary gain and not as they really are: organisms of the Mystical Body nourishing its wounded cells.

God wants man to use his environment primarily for his welfare. God helps man through nature. And one of nature's aids is the medical profession, men and women blessed by God with acuity and dexterity for the science of medicine and surgery. But even in the pages of history, the medical profession as well had to establish itself honorably. Before such a foreshadowing could attain practical significance, however, medicine had first to dispel the fog of superstition and error that shrouded illness and disease. It had to replace ignorance and fear with sound knowledge. God and man had to work together.

With the maturity and growth of scientific investigation, medicine has, thank God, recently developed new viewpoints and practices. One important viewpoint is the *emphasis on prevention*. In accord with this purpose, medicine offers, for example, vaccination and immunization injections besides recommending sanitary and other health measures. It also urges us to prepare and eat nutritious diets, control our weight, and visit our doctor periodically for health check-ups. What we are stating here is the practice of the theological virtue of temperance: the use of God's gift of reason over our lives. God is the Author of life, and we by His commandments (Thou shalt not kill) are urged to take care of ourselves without reckless behavior.

Another recent development in medicine is the growth of specialization. For example, obstetricians deliver babies, pediatricians safeguard the newborn through childhood, geriatricians care for those in their senior years. Then there are the allergists, gynecologists, eye specialists, ear, nose, and throat specialists, cardiologists, orthopedists, as well as general practitioners. So, all together, and with teamwork, these medical men and women have with God's grace produced healings. They have prolonged life, prevented disease, alleviated pain, performed surgery, effected cures. God indeed works through these human agents.

Called unto the Power to Heal

Healing is a power that belongs to God. All healing is of God alone. Man can heal no one. Man can only help the process of nature, as does the noble profession of the physician and surgeon. Man can help one to release his faith, which is a condition for healing, not its cause. The cause is God, through the agent the Holy Spirit. This concept is one that is very often misapplied, to the detriment of many a simple person. So often intense, agonizing pain of guilt is inflicted by ignorance in some who would appropriate a healing ministry! What a terrible tragedy to a human person to make him think that God has no care for him due to quantitative lack of so-called faith. God is the Healer through His mercy and love. When God uses those whom He wills to use so as to help a person return to health at some level of his or her being, then that person being ministered to is experiencing the gift of healing. It is a supernatural gift of God given by God Himself to a person. It flows from God's pure heart of mercy and love directly to the affected illness as a primary end, and then to a spiritual renewal of soul, which is the ultimate end of the healing.

When God imparts healing, as I perceive it, He is doing so as His personal expression of His concern motivated by His love. Since it is a gift, we can use it as we wish. But the intent of God is that through the healing we will arise to a new expression of behavior in accord with the Christian gospel. Through healing, God may be giving an individual some added time, be it a month or a year or two, solely that the individual may refocus his views toward the "great healing."

Divine healing, as I repeatedly state, is accomplished by faith in God, the Healer, Who can and Who will heal. Without the *condition* of faith, medication can be ineffective. Without faith, one who prays for another's healing is helpless. Jesus said: "As you have believed so be it done to you." (Mt. 8:13) One's believing must be a definite act of faith in God. (see Mt. 9:27–29)

When God calls a person to the healing mission, it appears that God is summoning this individual to "full surrender" of his whole

being and existence. When one is authentically called to the vocation of the healing apostolate, such a one is also enriched with the
tool for healing: *the power of prayer*. In the healing administration,
both he who is called as channel for healing and those called to be
prayed with for healing are sensitized through the power of prayer to
the presence of God.

For those who pray for healing, I have observed over and over
again a twofold distinction that actually and factually takes place.
At some prayer groups, healing takes place occasionally. The reason is
that perhaps the personality of that particular prayer group is not a
healing one but has another distinctive personality, such as derived
from one or more of the other charismatic gifts. It could be one of
love, one of prophecy, one of discernment, etc. However, this does
not mean that the other gifts are not present and not at work. It appears that all the gifts will eventually be present in the prayer group
as it develops in time and in maturity. On the other hand, as in my
own ministry, the distinctive personality is that of healing. And
within its sessions many other beautiful charismatic gifts are manifested in the other members serving in their respective capacities as
well as in me. How beautiful God's presence is among us!

The power to heal has many effects on the whole person. Some of
these healing effects are quite perplexing, especially if they are true
miracles. Others pertain to psychosomatic ailments, spiritual needs,
emotional or sociological problems, etc. And so any healing effect—
be it in the realm of authentic miracle (like blindness restored or vision imparted to one born blind, or neurological diseases healed),
psychological cure (emotional disturbance overcome, interpersonal
relationship renewed), physical restoration (including psychosomatic
disorders as asthma or ulcers, etc.), or spiritual restoration (one's
soul renewed in the presence of the Almighty by restored faith,
hope, and love, by a recommitment to a moral, upright discipline)—
accents the fact that the healing power of the Lord is present. But
be these healing effects what they may, as we are prone to categorize
them for analytical purposes, nevertheless it is the power of the
prayer used which removes the impediments. As these are removed,
restorative power for healing transmits itself throughout the sick person *holistically*.

It is necessary that one perceive intelligently that healing effects
are not to be expected simply because it may be medically desirable.

They are expected because the Word of God and his servant needs to be authenticated and illustrated. I personally do not consider my healing mission as a primary purpose for healing manifestations. But through the healing gifts, actual visible signs, the purpose of evangelization is dispersed to the broken body of the Church. One can see the logic in these thoughts. Primary and above all else is one's true vocation; all else is secondary, steps at the most, powerful as they may be, to the main purpose of one's summoning. One can moreover perceive that the fringe of the area of the new evangelization on the mission fields is very powerful; and it would be the most likely spot for miraculous healings to occur. One need only read the factual accounts of crusades by all denominations who present a program of evangelization to the poor and the sick in those lands most destitute. In these forsaken areas of the Third World, miracles and all other sorts of healings are numerous and can least be proved scientifically. The simple faith of the people at times can put to shame the cerebral.

PART II

Faith, Hope, Love

Most Christian teaching about healing places a strong emphasis on the role of FAITH. This message of FAITH is a needed and a true teaching. Jesus invites us to stand on His promises and claim our full inheritance as His brothers and sisters. However, an emphasis on FAITH that neglects the roles of LOVE and HOPE is unbalanced. We need to see all three aspects of the Gospel of Jesus Christ—FAITH, LOVE, and HOPE—and apply them all when speaking of healing.

Faith for healing helps us focus on the POWER of Christ (see 1 Co. 12:4–11) so that when we pray for healing, we should pray with the attitude of expectant FAITH knowing that Christ, in His POWER and LOVE, comes to us. ". . . come, Lord Jesus!" (Rv. 22:20) It is the LOVE of the Father for the Son and the Son for His Father and their LOVE for each other, called Spirit, that gives us an example of the DIVINE COMMUNITY on which all human relationships are built.

It is this LOVE that heals the total person. This LOVE, when expressed in our daily lives, heals. To nurture and to care for another heals gradually, and it is an expression of Jesus' love. To repent, heals; to forgive self and others, heals; to receive the Eucharist, heals; to be anointed, heals; to unbind ourselves from inner hurts and longtime wounds, heals. An understanding of healing based on LOVE emphasizes the character of Christ.

Hope balances both our FAITH and our LOVE. Hope is a firm expectation that God the Father will give us what He promises. His Son, Jesus, came to give us abundant, eternal life.

We have that life now and yet its full glory awaits His coming and our resurrection. (see Jn. 11:25–26) We have only the first fruits of the Spirit now (see Rm. 8:23), a foretaste of the glory that will be revealed. It is in that context that we administer healing, and it is in that context that healing is always a MYSTERY, a MYSTERY of HOPE. We do not know why some suffer more than others, nor why some are healed and others are not. We do know that God's ultimate goal is to bring us to wholeness and that the suffering of this present time is not worth comparing with the glory that is to be revealed to us. (Rm. 8:18)

Forgiveness, the Foundation of Healing

A basic foundation for healing is *forgiveness.* Jesus Himself, from the cross, proclaimed openly as He was hanging there: "Father, forgive them; they do not know what they are doing." (Lk. 23:34) After this word proclaimed from the cross, Jesus accepted the internal anguish of the thief who became good and, through forgiveness, offered him healing, reconciliation, righteousness, regeneration, rebirth.

By way of elaboration, I was once conducting a service in Shrewsbury, Massachusetts. God allowed me, through the Word of Knowledge (God indicating to me that within the assembled body a certain effect of healing love was being factualized) to identify a gentleman who was being healed holistically. He had been afflicted with an illness that consigned him to crutches. He screamed during the service, as a bolt of lightning (according to his description) had penetrated his body. Crying copiously, he rose to his feet and hobbled over to me, still holding on to his crutches but not truly walking on them. I addressed him: "You seem healed from your affliction. Are you experiencing at this moment any pain?" With tears flowing from his eyes, his mouth enunciating muffled words due to his crying, he mumbled, "No!" I then asked him if he felt that he could walk without the use of crutches, which he was holding very casually. I asked him if he would walk forward, and he did for a few paces. Again I questioned him: "Are you experiencing any pain?" With some consciousness of what was taking place in the moment, he more composedly enunciated, with greater force, a loud "No! No pain." Again I questioned him: "Were you undergoing any pain when you came to the service?" He answered that he had been in excruciating pain. He then dropped the crutches. There was no pain. He stood erect and upright, but as he walked forward he still hobbled. I knew that the physical healing was taking place but there was still in his spirit another attachment to some force or block that was impairing the complete healing. I questioned him with caution but firmness: "May I ask you a personal question?" He replied: "Yes, please do." (There were three or four hundred people present in that assembly.) Though I knew what the answer would be, I gently inquired: "Have you had an argument with someone recently?" With amazement his eyes beamed, his mouth opened and with tears again being resurrected profusely, he cried forth: "Yes!" I still questioned further, for his inner soul was being peeled to expose his ego and his need. "May I ask you more questions?" He replied with a tonality of surrendering himself completely to whatever I would ask: "Yes." I asked the final sensitive question: "Do you hate that person?" Bombastically he shouted with a desire to reconcile his harbored hatred: "Yes, my wife. She has left me and she divorced me." Consolingly, I further questioned him with a gentle direct approach: "You would like to forgive her now, wouldn't you?" As he wanted to forgive, he nevertheless had to burst forth his last cry of hatred for the hurt she had caused: "I hate the _____ but . . . I forgive her." Smilingly, after hearing the noun that he had used to describe his hatred, which is censored from this written narration, I offered the realization of his substantial healing: "You have no longer any pain, have you?" The reality of the moment overpowered him with its positive concreteness. He shouted to the aroused audience: "No. No. The pain is all gone. I'm healed." And he ran up and down the aisle to the affirmative applause of those who witnessed not only a physical manifestation of a man's restoration but a spiritual renewal, release of emotional accumulation, the proclamation of his sin now before the Lord, receiving pardon. He was totally healed as he gave up the hatred that was festering within him. He was brought to forgiveness and received pardon from Him who has power to forgive. *Forgiveness is the foundation of healing.*

Inner Healing

Another interesting insight in the healing ministry is that when we pray for the alleviation of a symptom we must go beneath that symptom to the ultimate cause of the problem. For example, during one of my services a little child was brought to me from the audience after I had identified his illness of asthma. One who is trained in holistic medicine knows that asthma, though it be organic in its condition, is only a symptom of a deeper, underlying problem or situation. When one prays for the removal of asthma, he is only praying for alleviation of the symptom, but this is not the basic approach to a complete healing. The underlying causative factor of the asthmatic attacks, at least for a child, would be environmental fears threatening his security. With this particular child who approached me for a prayer for healing from his asthma, I was friendly, bearing within my own mind the thinking process of a child. I pretended to question him. The questions served a twofold purpose: to relieve the child of his anxiety and to serve as introspection for healing the minds and the hearts, the attitudes and dispositions of his parents, who accompanied him. So the first question I asked the child was "Do you have asthma?" "Yes," responded the little boy. With a smile that served to further his ease, I paused briefly before going on. "How are Mommy and Daddy doing?" "Okay." His eyes, his mien, his tone of voice spoke to me more enlighteningly about the situation than his laconic verbal reply. Then I asked, utilizing a more delicate tone in my own voice while I sensitively probed a deeper nerve of this child's problem: "Do Mommy and Daddy always speak nicely?" The little boy's eyes opened and he blurted forth: "Daddy sometimes says something different to Mommy. They fight a lot." Immediately I recognized the cause that had to be treated for the healing of this boy's asthmatic attacks. Ruminating within the imagination of this little youngster was the threat of divorce, of separation, of being left alone. That was his basic concern.

He reminded me of the little boy who went up to his father and said, "Daddy, what happens to all the little boys whose mommy and daddy die in the United States? His father gave him statistics. But the child, attempting not to disclose his insecurity further, probed the father's mind and questioned, "Daddy, what happens to the little boys whose mommy and daddy die in the state of Minnesota?" (He and his family live in Minnesota.) And again Daddy gave him the statistics. "But, Daddy," the boy questioned further and with greater emphasis: "What happens to a little boy if his mommy and daddy die in our little city of Duluth, Minnesota?" Then the father realized what his son was really asking: Daddy, if you and Mommy continue to argue and fight, what happens to me if you and Mommy divorce?

For this reason, we must consider basic causes of sickness when we pray for diseases. Some sicknesses return because the entire healing process was not properly, not adequately, not intelligently completed. This is also the essence of inner healing.

Inner healing is a powerful and tremendous tool for the restoration of spirit, soul, and body. In essence, the dynamics of inner healing are nothing else but the psychological and spiritual processes of unpeeling an onion of its layers of skin—slowly, cautiously, prudently, with much respect for time elapsing. It is living an incident of our past lives, be it conscious or unconscious, resurrecting that wound with the presence of the love of Jesus, Who, through His own wounds, nurses us unto a resurrected, conscious dealing with that memory. The basic power of God's presence in that healing is the grace of forgiveness—being forgiven as well as forgiving another, being loved and loving another as Jesus would forgive and as Jesus would love us and that other.

Inner healing, which deals with our emotions and psychological problems, appears to be the most needed of healings. This form of healing corresponds with the depth insights of contemporary psychology, which holds in essence that our present condition has its roots in the formative years of our being. That is why we do inner healing through tracing the stages of life, of growth, because somewhere along the line there is something there causing our present behavior to be as it is. By going back and resurrecting the past properly, intelligently, with hope through prayer, we are able to bring it out onto the conscious level. We can then recognize it and we no longer need to escape it. We can handle it, we accept it, and we forgive. We ask Jesus to go to the wound that we experienced and heal it. Then we are free.

The basic step to inner healing is to relive the wound with Christ. Christ is the Wounded Healer for us who are wounded seekers. When we ask Jesus to go back with us to those incidents in our lives that have frightened us, we ask Him in humility to *transform*, not to throw the memories away. Then we are able to look back at them in peace. Through the healing power of God, they have lost their power to hurt us. This is psychological healing, called the healing of memories.

Many of our sessions, especially in smaller assemblies exposed to the weekend retreat with an atmosphere of prayer and silence, have offered these healing blessings. The healing of memories is a very delicate tool of spiritual psychology. It should not be utilized by the neophyte. It should be utilized in the hands of the professional, the intelligent, the prudent, the prayerful, and the humble. One's main concern is never to hurt another human being. It should also be cautioned, for the love of God and the love of people, that those blessed with inner healing should not be imitated by those who may desire to practice healing as a demonstration of charismatic expression. Psychiatrists and psychoanalysts appropriate the analogy of the onion as they deal in the realms of the human psyche. In the dynamics and processes of analysis, the onion is peeled gently, cautiously, layer by layer, until through the process of time, insight, association, reaction, transference, the healthy goal of resurrecting the true ego is achieved. One has thus touched the core of the human personality. The peeling of the layers has reference to the years lived by the client or the patient or the one seeking healing. These years vary: seven, ten, fifteen, twenty, seventy-two, eighty-four years. We must proceed tactfully, according to the pace that the client or the patient or the person seeking healing can tolerate. One must never imprudently or abruptly strike the nerve of the problem until all things are considered and adequately present themselves for such sensitivity. That's what psychological healing is all about.

Inner healing is extremely time-consuming, due to the distinctiveness of each case that is presented. One must be ever cautious in dealing with the mind, psyche, and soul. Some cases require many months and perhaps even a year or more in order that an adequate restoration of life be made. Many wonderful people suffer illnesses that are psychosomatic. Some are even paralyzed and experience actual organic ulcerations within their system. Other souls experience profound and deep spiritual destitution. There truly is a spiritual death in many souls who have not yet closed their eyes to this world. And as they grow older and years of experience accumulate, their subconscious mind is crying for emergence, for balm, healing.

Many people have come to us after having been spiritually dead, away from all forms of healthy religious behavior and practice, for thirty-five or even fifty years. They come to us with eyes that must cry tears of emptiness, separation, loneliness, borderline despair. What are some of the things they actually fear losing? The answer to this question bears within itself the element and process for healing. We who are called to serve these seeking souls must equip ourselves by prayer and knowledge. With a life of prayer and knowledge, we can confidently help these people to unfold and to resurrect their inner fears, perplexities, destitutions.

One of the first and basic steps toward uncovering people's problems is to aid them to resurrect and to handle their emotion of hate. Many people who have been hurt in life seek to retaliate with their emotion of hate. Years pile upon years. Feelings of revenge continue to mask themselves, mingling with further figments of the imagination. And the person never seems to unbind the other person, who has hurt him or her, and the one to suffer is the very person hating. Psychic energies starved from spiritual insight and prayer turn upon themselves. Sickness and disease ensue. Some of this hate, which has internalized itself in reverse, can also produce cancer. According to medical statistics, much of the cancer that is diagnosed today has its origin in the inappropriate use of the emotion of hate. Our duty as channels of healing must be to pray and to intercede that the roots of hate be removed.

Another interesting element of concern in the process of healing persons internally is the uprooting of guilt. There are countless persons who travel their lives in anxiety, overburdened with feelings of false guilt. A consoling thought for those who struggle with guilt and for those who may help another conquer guilt is that not all guilt is from God. Guilt feelings might come from certain social systems, or may be a product of unselected and unhealthful reading. On the other hand, guilt might be real. At other times it might not be real. However, if a person is feeling guilt, let that person ask himself: "Did I really feel this wrong thing? Did I willingly do this wrong thing? Did I wholeheartedly, without reservation, intend to do it?" If his response to all three questions is yes, then let that person say, "I am sorry, and I will start again."

Still another causative factor for much physical sickness and emotional disturbance, even spiritual destitution and immaturity, focuses around worry. I have addressed this theme to many of my audiences who have attended my retreats and spiritual renewal sessions. The cries of these people in pain are almost incredible. Fear, too, is an area of concern that takes its toll on people's bodies and minds, with its multiple forms of symptomatic expression.

If one is going to serve people properly in such a ministry as this, then the dynamics of what is taking place in the bodies and minds of people who come for healing must be appropriately understood and delicately unraveled. Our ministry exposes us to many persons who are of the golden age. In dealing with such, we are confronted with a host of attitudes that are subconsciously opposing the healing process. They serve staunchly as a block to healing. One of the basic attitudes of people who have reached old age is pain born of a sense of rejection. The fear of rejection reigns supreme among this group. And be it real or imaginary, to them it is important. A tool or mechanism of defense used to conquer rejection is self-pity, nurtured by the elderly person's enslavement of other people. Deep within themselves lurks subconsciously the desire to be accepted. The tool of this desire to obtain recognition, concern, and care is sickness. I say this with all due respect to the elderly, many of whom come to healing services that are being held in every parish of every city, all across the land. Consciously they state that they want to be healed, but subconsciously, for many, illness is desired as a means to hold on to that last hope of human affiliation. Although they wish to be healed, for no man wants illness, within themselves there is a psychic force that rejects healing virtue. The human psyche is very tricky in its self-defenses. To be healed may actually restore independence. It may mean the severance of a nursing daughter, of an overpossessed son, a husband's pitiable attention. It may even soothe the sick person's guilt for having offended the one who now nurses him. We have acutely noticed that some people, especially within certain ethnic groups, will not separate themselves from their canes even if they are healed objectively and authentically. To be healed would separate them from their internal enslavement to self-interest, self-seeking attention, and the service they receive from others.

There was a young girl to whom our ministry had been exposed by the process of healing. She was a fine young lady but with some deep-seated situations of life that caused her much mental pain. She pretended to be sick in order to acquire attention. She even used sickness to obtain subsidy from the government. Insight, caution, prudence, and prayer offered her the fruits of the dynamics of the deliverance ministry. By process and in time she was liberated from her guilty dependency.

Another shocking story that I often relate is that of a daughter whom I knew who attended and nursed her crippled mother for twenty years. The mother had been bedridden. Emotionally possessed by her mother, the daughter sacrificed many an opportunity of vocation and a status of marriage in order to take care of her invalid mother. One day as the daughter was going to take a day off, she said to her mother: "Mom, I'm going to go away for the day. I need to relax." She left the house, but soon remembered that she had forgotten something. She came back home, unannounced. As she walked by her mother's bedroom she thought she would open the door to peek in quietly so as to assure herself that the poor invalid mother was resting comfortably. As the door opened gently and quietly, she suffered a traumatic shock. There before the daughter's eyes, walking to and fro across the floor, was her mother, smoking a cigarette. The mother had pretended to be sick for twenty years. She did this to hold on to her daughter. That daughter left that house, never to return again. She went away aged, bitter, broken, and with hatred. What a price some psychic disturbances exact from the minds of men.

And so these are some of the people that we in the healing apostolate meet. The lives of others may always remain as strangers to us. One may never objectively know what other people are undergoing: their suffering, their hurt, their doings, their living.

What does it mean, then, to restore a person to health? One's immediate thought races itself to the concept of physical health. All healing is not to be considered merely physical. People vary according to personality, individual traits and distinctions, temperaments, culture, and nationalities. People become sick holistically, and one of the most important areas—in fact the miracle of healing—is that of healing the spirit. Man's spiritual life relates itself to His Creator, God. Sometimes people offend God; sometimes people even hate God. Actually, people really don't hate God; that which they hate is the circumstances that they have undergone painfully and that they think God should have changed.

Hatred has many faces. If we depict it, its foolishness—although important to us at that moment—can be very embarrassing. For example, we have heard people say: "God, I hate you. I hate you for making me be born an Italian. I hate you, God, for making me French or Irish. I hate you, God, for allowing me to lose my job. I hate you, God, for this grotesque body you have given me; for making me short, chubby, freckled. I hate you, God, for the man you made me marry." Well, God didn't make you marry that man, or that woman. What is happening is that one is reacting to something one cannot control; and so, reverting to childhood attitudes and traits, one screams and yells as a reaction and retaliation. Sometimes one may utter that one hates one's wife or husband, but objectively it is not hate of the spouse that he or she is experiencing. One does not hate a sinner. What one is experiencing is anger toward that type of behavior.

Our Blessed Lord Himself teaches that one must not hate the sinner. One is to hate the sin. In so dealing with the emotions in psychological healing, one is working with the eleven passions: love, hate, sadness, joy, pleasure and pain, fear and boldness, desire and aversion and anger. These are good emotions. God gave them to us. But these emotions can disperse themselves in many ways. God gives us His grace to recognize, control, and direct these powers. He gives us the virtues of fortitude, justice, love, and temperance. It is in the realm of our reasoning and ascetical life to control the emotional reactions pertaining to the pros and cons of life.

A word of insight for those who deal with the spiritual direction of souls may be interesting here. The vocation of one called to such direction is not only of high esteem but must be borne with conscious responsibility. His qualities must be those of an authentic director of souls; namely, technical and moral. One called to direct another man's life must submit himself or herself as well as direct the counselee to the ordinary workings of Divine Providence. The dynamics utilized for spiritual direction are founded in the art of leading souls progressively from the beginning of the spiritual life to the height of Christian perfection. Being an art, it is therefore a practical science. Its nature rests upon the guidance of supernatural prudence as applied to a particular case. Whatever the case may be, the director who seeks and leads a soul in search of God enriches that person with the principles of the theology of Christian perfection. As in other sciences of maturity, so in Christian growth, the orientation to Christian living must be done progressively, that is, according to the strength and need of the soul being blessed at that given moment. The prudence of applying direction to another human person is thus given with responsibility as soon as that soul is definitely resolved to travel. Hence the director fulfills validly his role as teacher, counselor, and guide.

The virtue of prudence is a condition without which the director of souls cannot function. Through him, right reason is applied to actions. Through him, the virtue of prudence enables a man to judge accurately what is the morally good thing to do under the particular circumstances encircling that soul. The virtue of prudence itself cannot be substituted by any other virtue, since it is essential to strong perfection. It not only enables a person to recognize and to discern, but it also directs him to avoid, evil. As it enlightens behavior with practical applicable insight, it also points out causes and occasions, opportune remedies, and the right judgment for each instance of human responsibility. One of the most torturous of human anxieties that can afflict the interior life of a human person is the loss of purpose for living. What a tremendous privilege is his or hers who, being utilized by God, directs another human person to the focus of his or her being. As soon as we have a purpose, we become straight. Is that not one of the goals of inner healing? In leading a soul to his or her purpose, one is also enriching that soul's power to love. Chesterton himself had proclaimed that to love each thing separately strengthens the power of loving. Or again, as Terence of old once uttered, nothing that is human can be foreign to us.

Noble indeed is that person blessed by God to direct a soul to inner peace and joy of spirit. By a journey within there comes forth a voyage of self-discovery through inscape. It is one of God's ways to heal the soul within. God walks into one's soul with silent steps. He comes to each soul more than the soul itself goes to Him. Many of the crosses we bear are of our own manufacture. A cross constructed by ourselves through God's love can place upon it the healing balm of Christ, the Divine Physician. Let each of us who are called to be channels of healing allow Christ to fill the vacuum of another person's life. He alone can make a human's life on earth a heavenly cathedral from the stable of his or her being. The greatest evil to threaten the advancement of a soul seeking union with God is self-love. God's healing touch is to produce a divesting of oneself . . . one's body, one's spirit, one's desires; our loves, our hates, our all.

No one is better because of pain. And when the inner self is enslaved to itself or to external agents controlling it, pain will result. Really a man suffering pain becomes seared and scarred by pain. The soul experiencing loneliness is exposed to the realities of the emptiness of itself. And that emptiness does drive that soul back into itself. God's grace for inner healing is then needed. If the human soul freely accepts that very emptiness produced by loneliness as a camouflaged grace of God, it then can grow to an additional plateau of self-sanctification, because it has cooperated with the divine grace of that moment. In that very instant, it radiates with smiles of joy in its completed voyage of discovery of the meaning of life.

As a sculptor utilizes the mallet and the chisel to produce his masterpiece upon the hardness and crudeness of a rock, so in the hands of the prudent and responsible internal healer is the power of inner healing—serving as an artistic chisel chipping away the internal tragedy of human anguish and pain. It is said that true sculptors see in their block of marble the statue of worth that they wish to create. In his work, the sculptor thus chips away on the block until just the finished figure of art remains. And thus, from the hand of inner healing, our lives are set free to perfection as we are chipped away, with our many flaws. Only the hand of the Divine Sculptor adds through life's experiences those things which are required for each one of us to realize our dream of personal betterment. Let the thoughts of Charles Dickens encourage those who have experienced inner healing to proclaim that whatever they have tried to do in life they have tried with all their hearts to do well.

Call to a New and Deeper Christian Life

When we experience the HEALING POWER and PRESENCE of Jesus' LOVE, we are filled with greater trust in Jesus. We have a deeper sense of HOPE in our future, because Jesus lives in us. When we have such an experience, the Lord Jesus is asking us to take on a new and deeper way of life. A new way of life means turning from wrongdoing (former ways of Godlessness) and accepting the Lord Jesus. A deeper way of life means living in a closer UNION with Father, Son Jesus, and Holy Spirit. All of us are expected to have Jesus first in our lives. All of us are called to be consciously aware of the Spirit of Jesus working in us, in others, and in creation. A new and deeper way of life calls us to a conscious belief that the Father plans every detail of our life for our good. A new and deeper way of life in Jesus is lived in loving service for our brothers and sisters. We are called to be at one with all God's people. "Father, may they be one in us, as you are in me and I am in you, so that the world may believe it was you who sent me." (Jn. 17:21)

Moreover, it is frequently noticed that when God offers a person healing, He is leading the soul to a new life of service. Perhaps this service can be likened to preventive medicine controlling the destructive forces of a person's life. To remember Jesus only when one is at the eleventh hour of his existence or in dire pain and then to forget him after being blessed, is a sad response to God's goodness. Through healing, God gives us added life to enrich our lives in the furtherance of our salvation. I have seen many people fall into worse conditions because they did not live the new life that Jesus gave them when He healed them. When we receive healing, it is like receiving a new life that does not belong to us. When Christ heals someone, that person is summoned to reconciliation, regeneration, righteousness, and rebirth.

It is often asked why not everyone is healed. I have spent many hours in prayer, in pondering this question. And though the paradox remains in our human understanding, yet the true answer remains a mystery. However, I have gradually come to conclude that it is not our avowed motives that hold back healings but the attitude dwelling behind our motives which is at fault. So often we are led astray by false assumptions that God can be glorified only by a witness of physical healing. And yet the objective truth remains that some people have made themselves saints by remaining in their chairs and beds of pain. Without their anguish, God could not speak to them. Without their pain, sanctified by the God who speaks with them, they could not become channels of redemptive intercessory prayer. Those of us who are authentically called and unselfishly serve in valid apostolates of healing have seen the light of Christ shine with ever more-blinding radiance in the eyes of those who suffer in His name and for His cause. It is also perceived that those who are thus blessed by grace to suffer redemptively are far more healthy than the individual blessed with physical health who yet remains spiritually dead. It is a greater blessing of God to glorify the Trinity when one must still suffer than it is to render Him honor and glory with more ease when one has received physical healing.

Faith produces hope. Hope ushers forth love. A community coming together in an atmosphere of prayer and devotion suddenly is transformed into an oasis of love. Life will always call for courage. Without it, we all become just playthings for life and may eventually realize that we are just humans. True love makes it possible for one to accept limitations. But genuine love is the most effective creator and promoter of human existence. All the world seems to be a stage of life for the great drama of love. But he who knows not life is he who knows not love, because life is a courtship between the soul and its Eternal Lover.

Prayer for Healing

Praying for physical healing is the simplest of the various forms of prayer. At the same time, it causes much anxiety, especially among the neophytes or the cerebrally inclined. Nevertheless, it is the *easiest* of prayers for healing. I think often of some of the instant and extremely dramatic healings that I have witnessed as well as others who have witnessed them with me: the man Leo Perras, paralyzed for twenty years, who walked; the teenager of St. Cloud, Minnesota, blind, who now sees; people with cancers of all sorts, now cured; men and women long deaf, now listening to the sonorous melodies of God's nature.

And so it is that prayer and prayer alone prepares both the individual and groups of individuals to become the receptive vessels for God's selective healings. Such prayer requires, as well as it prepares, an atmosphere of trust and faith for the community that has come together in the sharing of their broken humanity. Incidentally, it is for this reason that I prefer to conduct my mission of healing in assembled groups, rather than through private appointments. Nevertheless, God's grace of healing functions appropriately with each moment that He presents for healing prayer, be it private or public.

A faith-filled atmosphere conditions the audience to be receptive to healing love. A sense of holy expectation is engendered. One can almost sense its permeating influence as its Holy Spirit encircles

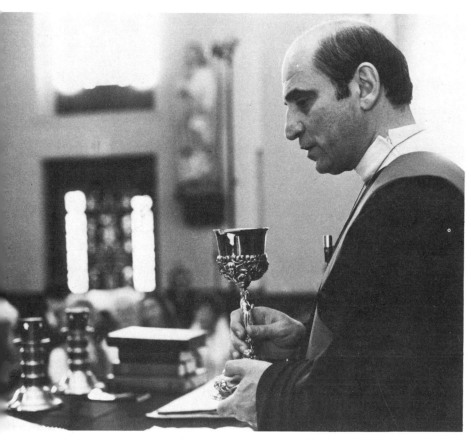

The heart of the service: Christ's presence among us brings peace and joy.

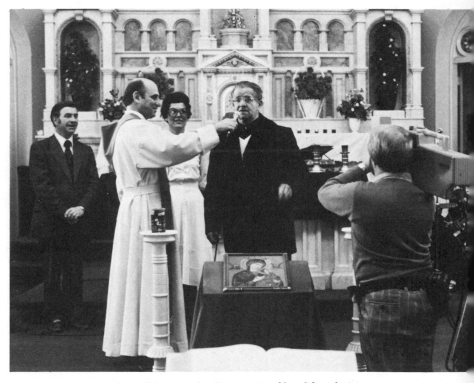

One of the many healing services filmed for television

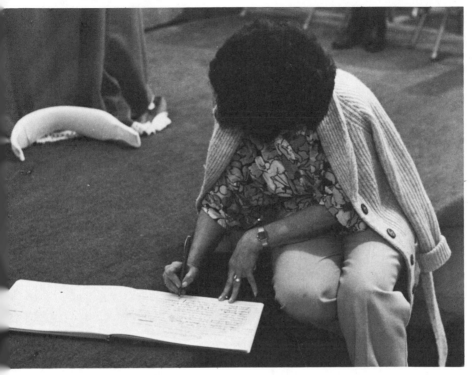

When a person claims a healing, it is recorded in a registration book. This book contains thousands of names and addresses.

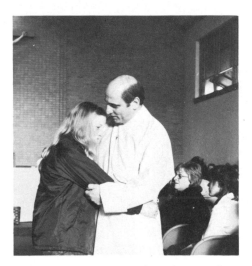
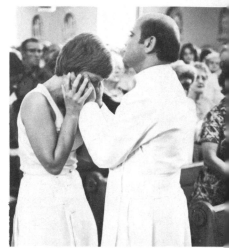

The embrace with compassion for inner healing

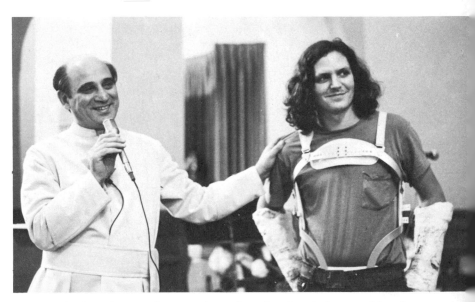

A total healing of injuries from an industrial accident; but the brace could not be removed at the time, because it was riveted on.

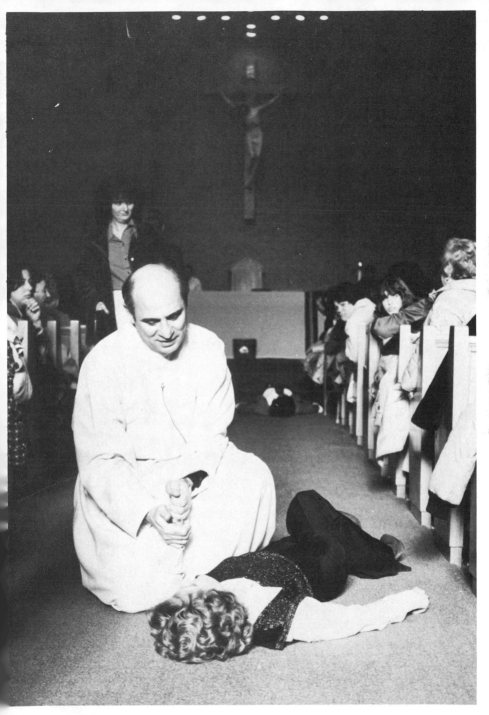

Most of the people prayed for are overpowered by the Holy Spirit.

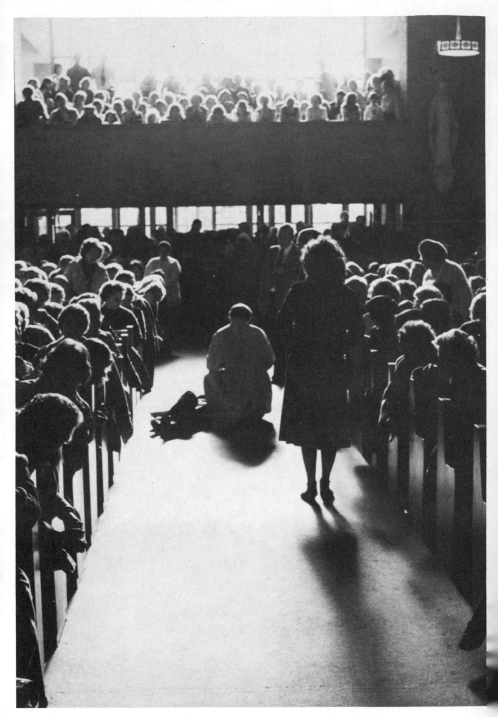

A rest in the peace of the Holy Spirit

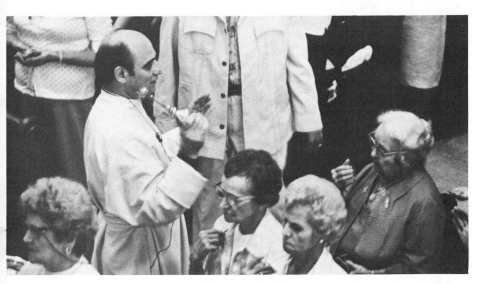

Prayer and blessings for all ages . . .

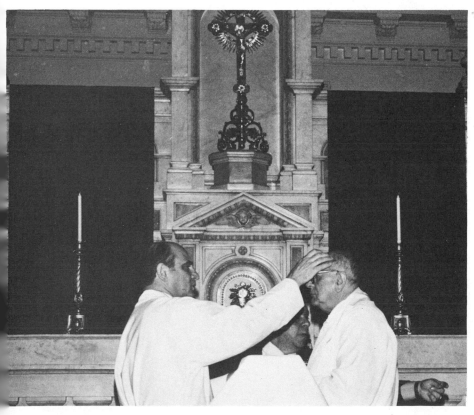

. . . and for fellow clergy

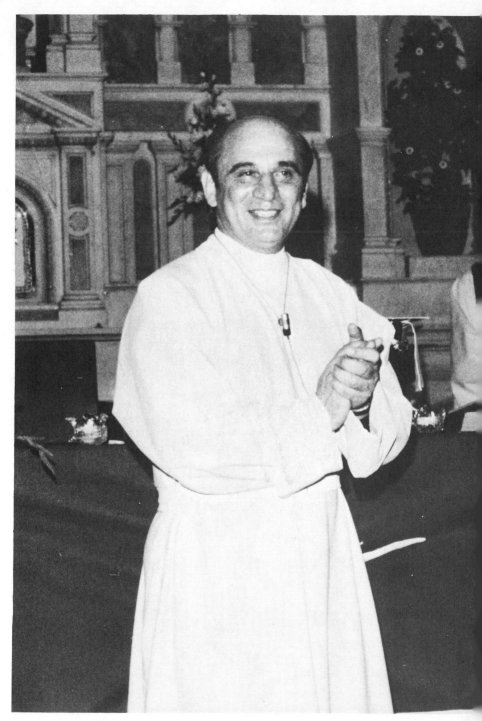

The joy of ministering to God's people

each and every one present. As one looks into the eyes of the sick, one can almost hear the facial expression emanating from the sick: "If he can walk out of that wheelchair, why can't I?"

As the spirit of love is born at a prayer service, as it is nurtured by the various ministries of that particular session, there spurts forth an incredible force of spiritual energies. If God emits these energies, we are, then, in the atmosphere and presence of divine healing love. As this love permeates and enriches the community of prayer, attitudes of all sorts become positive. There is forgiveness of sins; understanding between husbands and wives is experienced as never before. Nationalities and creeds find their identity and their oneness beneath Him who is their ABBA, their FATHER. Incredible as it may appear, that which wells up to the foe is the great communal expectation of human hearts wishing well—healing.

How should one pray for the sick? What type of prayer should be used? are questions frequently asked. When one talks to God, one should use the prayer book of one's own heart. No formulation, no special ritual can substitute for one's own interior experiences. Since humility (i.e., the recognition of human inadequacy) is the foundation from which God emanates His healing love, a cerebrally inclined person finds false security in his attempts at prayer. When one prays for physical healing as well as inner healing, one should be positive; one's prayer should center itself on health and upon the healing power of the divine cause of healing. It is necessary to zero in on the person of healing, Jesus Christ, and upon the agent of healing, the Holy Spirit. It is not necessary to focus on the disease, not to expend all our energies in healing prayer over the specific ailment. However, all things being involved, a conscientious healer determines the type of illness at hand. As he primarily speaks to the Lord in his healing prayer, he also incorporates the situation of illness presented through his intercessory power. By way of example, if one is dealing with depression, one is in the area of psychological disturbance. But, in the healing prayer, depression remains exactly what it is: namely, a symptom that is being gently treated but bypassed as soon as possible to deeper, underlying causes. One should not waste time with the symptom beyond that which is necessary, but cautiously, prudently, and gently journey within the causative factor—which in this case is anger. As anger is being dealt with through the process of inner healing, a further probing is undergone in order to expose the ultimate cause of the anger which has produced the symptom of depression and that is the lack of self-contentment, the real cause. With this insight, the healing prayer becomes an efficient tool in the healing process. With God's grace touching this natural process of psychoanalysis, one suddenly finds oneself endowed with the gift of divine healing, a true charism for the building up of a wounded soul.

What type of prayer should be used? We learn much from good example. We learn much from others, and so just as a doctor would consider the type of medicine to use in his treatment after his diagnosis, so those called to the healing mission should consider what type of prayer is most appropriate for the distinct situation at hand. Is it spiritual prayer? Is it psychological insight? Should family prayer be utilized? Is the prayer one for physical ailments? Is it one that belongs to the ministry of deliverance from obsessions? Is the situation at hand one that calls for the special prayer of exorcism?

Among the various categories of healing, deliverance holds a paramount position. It deals specifically with the forces of evil. Its dynamics involve the powers of exorcism over Satanic possessions and deliverance over demonic obsessions. As a remedy against these forces, prayer is applied. And it is objectively perceived that each illness can reflect upon the other. The prayers in turn should be appropriate to the illness. Spiritual and emotional illnesses dwell within the individual as they affect God and man's relationship (spiritual) and as they affect man with himself and with his interpersonal relationships (psychological). The physical devastations of man are produced by age, accident, and disease.

The Church herself, because of her wisdom throughout the ages, has brought forth formal ritualistic prayers for the needs of her people. The formulation of static prayers serves the purpose of retaining continuity and unison in prayer as made by the moral bond of unity existing in the praying community. The Church, moreover, has always sanctioned prayers and blessings against sickness, be they in the forms of preventive or curative intercessions.

History, too, has enriched our contemporary understanding of sickness and disease. And so today we use both preventive and curative prayer. Just as one would take preventive care of one's health by prudently watching the intake of proper food or by the utilization of hygienic measures, so does one pray to prevent illness. At other times, we are called to pray curatively. For example, if the person is already sick from disease, accident, or what have you, one would pray for the healing to commence as it proceeds to remove that which was diseased. Man has a tendency to look for an intercessor who would stand between the Almighty and the believer. People throughout the ages have found it pleasing though not absolutely necessary to turn to God's select and canonized intercessors, patron saints such as St. Camillus the healing saint, the popular St. Anthony, and the renowned St. Thérèse of Lisieux, praying for protection against particular diseases. Man in our day might utilize prayer meetings, crusades, and missions and turn to such gifted personages as Kathryn Kuhlman, Oral Roberts, myself, and many others who have been blessed with distinctive ministries, to intercede for healing.

To Pray as Jesus Did

The life of Jesus Christ was one of complete dedication to the Father's will. The prayer of Jesus informs us of His union with His Father throughout His life. His most difficult prayer came at the most trying time of His life, in Gethsemane. Realizing He was approaching His physical death, He prayed, "Father, if you are willing, take this cup away from me. Nevertheless, let your will be done, not mine." (Lk. 22:42) His prayer demonstrates how great is the mystery of the will of God the Father. We know that the Father reveals His will through Scripture, through the prophetic gifts, through our own time of prayer and meditation, and through the circumstances of life. Difficult as it may seem, Christian prayer is marked by a surrender to the Father's will in all things.

The Authentication of Healing

Although legitimate authority has discerned the ministry of prayer for healing as authentic and valid, proper respect remains due to those professions of medical attention and care for their valuable assistance and scrutiny. Zeal without prudence, neurotic emotional conclusions, must be strongly avoided. God, the Author of life and

the Provider and Sustainer, has introduced the medical profession to
deal with illnesses of the body and of the mind. God has endowed
men to be helpful to one another as man traverses the years of his
life. For illnesses that are organic or psychological in function, God
has created, out of the abundance of His healing compassion, men
and women acute and dexterous in their perception, scrutiny, diagnosis, and prognosis of such afflictions. Blessed are the hands of those
men and women called to minister to the wounds of afflicted humanity. For this reason—especially when the Apostolate of Prayer
for Healing relates itself to inner organic ailments or to internal
functional disorders of mind, such as metabolism or chemical im-
balances—a word of prudence is emphasized. Concerning those
afflicted persons experiencing healing of their natural diseases, we
urge that they present themselves to the medical profession for final
observation and diagnostic clarification. Thereupon the healing experience becomes objectively a true witness to supernatural intervention. If one believes that one has been authentically healed, or
that one's condition has been improved in some way, one must not
cancel one's doctor's appointments, nor should one stop taking one's
medication, nor should one refuse further treatment. God wills that
authentic channels of healing not only be respected but coalesce as
well into a unity of holistic oneness. In practice, therefore, one apparently healed must return to one's physician and under the doctor's diagnostic, scrutinizing eye have one's healing verified. This occasion can offer another splendid opportunity of witnessing and
enriching those called by God to be His hands and His mind, to be
His natural vehicle for healing power among men.

Healing and Evangelization

I hope by now that you have absorbed many practical and reflective concepts about the healing ministry. Many of the items
reflected upon are those which have been of paramount interest and
concern to those who bear a responsible commitment to the people
of God. It is so important to fathom the profundity of the truth
that any gift with which we may be endowed serves only as a stepping-stone!

In the Catholic Church there are two branches of evangelization:

One is called the propagation of the faith and the other the propaganda of the faith. Archbishop Sheen had been the Director of the Propagation of the Faith. Its purpose is to bring the faith, God's gospel and message, to a people who have never heard of the Lord Jesus Christ. It utilizes many programs and media. It subsidizes many missions and missionaries. It brings food and medicine and other necessities for the welfare of humanity. Through such programs of care, the minds and hearts of non-Christians and pagans are disposed to listen, to admire, to love, and to embrace the ways of the Good News. The Propaganda of the Faith, with which I associate my ministry, is an enriching of the faith. It is the spreading of evangelization to all the levels of humanity. The healing gift, with all its awesome manifestations, serves as a key that opens the door to the treasures of God's faith.

In the study of theology, there is a tract called *De Gratia*. This tract deals with God's grace, God's life. Within the contents of this treatise there is a statement: "In the course of man's life God will always give him 'sufficient grace' to know about Jesus Christ and to make a personal commitment to the Lord Jesus." This concept of "sufficient grace" is nothing else but God's promise to unveil Himself to humanity. In so doing, humanity in every phase would be confronted with the gospel message leading to a confrontation with oneself, to a moment of deliberation, and to a moment of decision to accept the Lord Jesus Christ as personal Lord and Saviour. When a person proclaims himself a sinner, as one in need, that person proclaims the Lord, and when he does so, the theology of sufficient grace produces the conversion. That moment of conversion transfers itself from sufficient grace to the efficient state of the new life.

When Father Pio was on earth, he had been blessed with many charismatic gifts. One of these manifesting gifts was that of the stigmata. Since the time of St. Francis of Assisi, who also experienced the stigmata, there was no other Catholic priest bearing such a gift. Father Pio was also well known for another charismatic gift: that of discernment. It was so powerful that in the process of his ministry, especially during confession, he could recognize sin or deceit. Many of the American GIs during the Second World War who were serving in the Allies' campaign throughout Italy have stated how Father Pio would read their consciences whenever they would come to him for guidance, counsel, or confession. All these external gifts, as well as the many external manifestations of this day, were and are extensions of Jesus' presence through a human channel of God's selection. Their sole purpose is to render to the human observers the person of Jesus.

The Healing Ministry

The purpose of the healing ministry is to invigorate the world that lies in anguish, that has lost hope. Through the healing manifestation, the lives of many people are brought to the Person of the Lord, Who revisits His people by bringing love back to the Church and the Church to love.

If one were to look in an index to the Scriptures, one would see the many listings pertaining to healing. I have cited some already. In Exodus 15:26, the Lord Himself proclaims Himself: ". . . for it is I, Yahweh, who give you healing." Farther on in the Scriptures one also reads, in 2 Ch. 7:14: ". . . then if my people who bear my name humble themselves, and pray and seek my presence and turn from their wicked ways, I myself will hear from heaven and forgive their sins and restore their land."

The world needs to be healed. The Scriptures leave for human posterity the example of King David, who, only after falling upon his knees and seeking God's forgiveness for his crimes, received a healing. It is narrated that King David in mid-life became a lonely man. As he wined and basked in his emptiness, he became ripe for the dissipation of an unhealthy sexual adultery. Bathsheba herself had been separated from her own husband, who was in the military service of the king and the government. This separation also made her ready for an affair. In the days that offered her loneliness and emptiness, as well as time for loitering, she made herself available to the king. These two dissipated souls brought themselves into unlawful unity. They had a child. Because of that adulterous sin, the king brought a disgrace both upon himself and upon his household. The hurt was severe and deep. The child died. The murder of Bathsheba's husband was added to the first sin. Sin has a way and tendency of adding to itself. Then the king's only son, Absalom, was killed. The king's conscience became agitated, disturbed. God sent the prophet Nathan to stir that restless conscience. Both the person of King David and his household needed to be healed. When David accused himself by his own words before the prophet Nathan, the ignominy and the magnitude of his sin brought tears to his eyes and sorrow to his repentant heart. As a penitent sinner he ripped his garments, fell upon his knees, and besought the Lord for mercy and renewed love. But notice, David comes forth renewed only when he falls upon his knees and cries: *Mea culpa, mea culpa, mea maxima culpa*—"through my fault, through my fault, through my most grievous fault." From that height of glory and honor he falls to the lowliness of sinful crime: From sinful lowliness he now is restored to the mercy of God and His love, to a higher state than ever before. Because of his fall, God, who draws good out of evil, was able to speak to David, to the king who now comes forth with the beautiful psalms of repentance. Within those psalms he proclaims how the brokenhearted are healed by God.

The book of Proverbs offers another beautiful source about healing, especially Proverbs 3:21–24: "My son, hold to sound judgment and to prudence, do not let them out of your sight; they will prove the life of your soul, an ornament around your neck. You will go on your way in safety, your feet will not stumble."

Jeremiah himself proclaims: "I will heal your faithlessness."

The book of Hosea narrates an impressive love story. It is the story of a faithful man close to God who was told by God to go and marry a harlot, a woman of the street, a prostitute. Out of her own spirit of insecurity, she one day leaves him, abandons him, goes forth to live her own life. But God retains Hosea as a special lover, true and loyal. The prostitute is drawn back home to Hosea. This woman is called Gomer and God heals her. She is a picture of Israel, whom God loves.

Luke, who was a doctor, a medical man, speaks and narrates, more than all the other writers of the Scriptures, about healings. His is a gospel for doctors and nurses to read, and reread, and meditate upon. The Acts of the Apostles and the letters to the Corinthians, speak adequately of the healings "by one spirit." St. James, in his Chapter 5, verses 14–15, offers the consolation of healing to the Christian community: "If one of you is ill, he should send for the elders of the church, and they must anoint him with oil in the name of the Lord and pray over him. The prayer of faith will save the sick man and the Lord will raise him up again; and if he has committed

any sins he will be forgiven." This exhortation of St. James is truly
spiritually uplifting and encouraging, as it offers the healing promise.
It speaks to one whose personal relationships may be strained. It
speaks to others whose emotions have gone astray. It rekindles one
whose body is diseased or who may be attacked by satanic forces.
Morever, it offers, to those suffering the effects of original sin and
to those who are dying, the healing presence of Christ, who wills to
call them unto wholeness of life.

In the previous reflections pertaining to healing, we have considered some very important things. Enough emphasis cannot be
placed on the fact that healing, in the Christian sense, means
healing of the whole person. When we minister healing in Christ's
name, we minister the whole of His redemptive love to the whole of
a person's being. Our Lord's redemptive work was to free humanity
from the total effect of sin, evil and ignorance.

In an attempt to consider some practical questions that are frequently presented to those of us who are involved in the healing
ministry, and in the hope that they will be helpful to you, I conclude with these summary reflections:

1. *What is divine healing?* There is much misunderstanding about
the healing ministry. The healing ministry presupposes pain. Within
man there is some kind of disorder emerging, from a common cold
to terminal cancer. Whatever it may be, mankind is engulfed in a
huge continuum of pain. Moreover, a plethora of human suffering
crowds the areas of our world: television programming, family life,
social and political events. The divine healing ministry in its essential concept is really to bring love back to the Church, and the
Church to love. It moreover invigorates the world, which lies in anguish. Divine healing is not a substitute for the doctor. God's
goodness to man incorporates the creation of medicine. To reject
medicine is to reject and deny the goodness of God. Divine healing
is not Christian Science. Jesus did something about pain and illness.
He accepted the reality of disease. Jesus never brushed aside illness
and disease as though it were the product of one's mental outlook.
Instead, from Scripture we read how He overpowered such sickness
and disease with His compassion, mercy, and healing love. Jesus
Himself was no stranger to suffering, and because of this He under-

stands, appreciates our pain, loves us, and heals us. Moreover, His Church walks in His footprints, seeking to alleviate pain by its many institutions and charitable organizations such as Catholic Relief Services. Divine healing is not faith healing. It is tragic to hear people state that perhaps the reason they are not healed is because they lack enough faith. As I continually stress, healing from God does not depend upon our quantitative faith or upon our good works. God's gift of healing flows completely from the mercy and love of His bountiful goodness. Divine healing is not even positive thinking, though positive attitudes are important in healing. Doctor Michael Snyder, at St. Vincent's Hospital in Worcester, has worked with patients who claim that they have been healed of cancer through the prayers of our own ministry of the Apostolate of Prayer for Healing. Doctor Snyder is quoted as saying in regard to the healing services of prayer how they are of positive benefit to the healing process of the sick:

> They give people much needed hope, a positive approach to life during a very difficult stage. They offer faith and support, which helps place the patient in the proper frame of mind for therapy. I'd say they play an important role as long as they don't interfere with the treatment process, as long as their role is kept within its proper perspective.

Positive thinking sometimes makes the difference between living and dying. Positive thinking does not offer the power to save a soul. The ministry of healing is ultimately involved with the salvation of the whole man. Divine healing includes a person's relationship to God. Divine healing is not the momentary relief from pain. Many Christians are nominal Christians. Many Christians, as long as they are healthy and secure for a short period of time, do not give much concern to God. When they fall sick, many rush to the Lord. Christians must be careful not to use religion or Christ as a hot-water bottle or a Band-Aid, taking him off the shelf when we hurt and putting Him back when the pain is gone.

2. *What is a healing service?* There is common agreement that if two or more gather together in prayer and call upon the Lord, God is in their midst. And so a healing service is the administration of divine healing love for the one purpose of attending to, caring for,

and praying with an individual or group of people who desire healing
in body, mind, and spirit for themselves or for others. And during
such sessions where the people are gathered together, the people's
faith is nourished with the promises that are read in Scripture. The
Word is preached, confession of sins is proclaimed, absolution and
forgiveness are pronounced, prayer is intently offered, and for those
who belong to a sacramental church, the sacraments are enjoyed. At
other times, the directive of St. James is utilized and the anointing
with oil is carried on; sometimes there is the laying on of hands.
Prayers for the sick have always been most precious to both God,
Who hears, and to the people, who pray. At still other times during
a session for healing, especially in smaller groups, an opportunity
for counseling, guidance, and spiritual direction is had. Such services
of healing can be held anywhere: in private sessions, huge audi-
toriums, churches, homes, and among the family members themselves.

3. *What is the relationship of divine healing to the medical profession?* In considering ways in which healing is administered in the
Church, it is appropriate to mention the medical profession. "Honor
the doctor with the honor that is his due in return for his services;
for he too has been created by the Lord. Healing itself comes from
the Most High, like a gift from a king." (Si. 38:1–2) There need be
no conflict between divine healing and the medical profession. If I
cut my finger, the blood will in time coagulate and gradually the
flesh will knit together and the cut will be healed. This is because
the body has natural healing resources given to it by God. A doctor
acts to facilitate the natural healing powers of the body. The same
can be said of the surgeon and the psychiatrist. The latter's purpose
is to help the patient realize his condition and its cause and gain
his cooperation to release inherent resources and so enable him
again to embrace life.

In all of this it is the God-given healing powers of the body and
personality that operate. The medical profession is following God's
laws even if members of it repudiate Him and some of their
methods and attitudes are questionable. Where there is cooperation
with the medical profession, the result is of great benefit to those
who suffer.

In one of my parishes it was my good fortune to have a few Christian doctors with whom I could work closely. This gave us the opportunity to discuss people in need. Their medical knowledge often proved invaluable to me and they accepted and used my ministry. We found this mutually encouraging and enlightening, and we had the satisfaction of knowing that our combined knowledge and personal gifts, dedicated as they were to Christ, ensured that those whom we served were receiving from us the best we had to give. One of the doctors was a psychiatrist, and so, together, we were able to offer Our Lord's healing on all three levels: spirit, mind, and body.

This happy arrangement does not, I am sure, exist everywhere. There can be on both sides distrust, ignorance, and sometimes downright criticism, but such attitudes may be broken down and co-operation encouraged. Since the medical profession is fast moving away from its former concentration on the physical aspect of healing and is realizing the part that spirit and mind play in the life and health of people, there is hope that from their side cooperation with the Christian ministry will increase. And conversely, clergy and ministers should demonstrate to doctors that they have a power for healing from Christ that they can offer.

4. *Why are not all healed?* Any valid healing ministry must face this baffling question. We do not always see "signs and wonders." WHY? Answer: I do not know. There is no easy answer to the problem of suffering. It will always remain a mystery, centered in the Cross. Once, I laid hands on a woman who had cancer and she received an immediate healing. A year later, she became sick with another ailment; namely, a fever and an infection. Again I prayed with her, but the infection took its full course and she received apparently only the blessing of the Spirit. Why was there healing in the first instance and not in the second?

Cases like this are puzzling, and we must face the fact that such experiences occur in the healing ministry. It is definitely difficult to explain these things. All that we can do is to place ourselves as fully as possible in Our Lord's hands.

There are many factors that inhibit healing. For example, the sick person may not be ready for ministry either emotionally or as regards faith in God. If so, the Holy Spirit does not lead us to pray for healing. Some people still believe that God sends suffering either to purify or to punish. How often people say, "It's my cross" or "I am a wicked man. I deserve this."

Another major reason for the lack of healing is that large numbers of Christians still do not believe that Christ will heal. Others have reservations of different kinds: While large numbers of Christians believe that Christ *can* heal, they have not sufficient faith to believe that He *will* heal. Such a burden of doubt has to affect our ability to receive the healing love of Jesus. FOR THIS REASON IT IS VERY IMPORTANT THAT CLERGY INSTRUCT THEIR CONGREGATIONS.

Sometimes there is unrealized or unrepented sin, or an unwillingness to forgive. When praying for healing in the emotional life, and in some cases one has to reach deeply to an unexposed hurt, it may be that the person concerned cannot yet bear to look at what has been such a shattering experience, and so healing will be delayed. Also, the cause of the difficulty may be demonic, rather than physical or emotional (the deliverance ministry is special and unique).

These things that I am mentioning should serve to indicate that the ministry of healing is not necessarily straightforward. Many factors are involved. Should there not be an immediate healing, we therefore need not be discouraged. Jesus told us to persevere by asking, seeking, and knocking. (Lk. 11:5–10)

In spite of these difficulties, we should continue to pray for the healing, lay on hands, and even anoint with oil as many times as may be necessary. And as we do, we should ask the Holy Spirit to reveal the blockages. Where healing is administered "in an honest and good heart," God always acts to bless. Difficulty should not let us lose heart, but on the contrary, force us into a closer life with Christ.

Although this chapter may be quite long, one must realize that such a vast subject as healing is extremely complex, as it is expansive. Within these concepts presented, I have dealt with areas of specific interest and concern for the better judgment of an authentic healing apostolate. I hope that these reflections have been of both interest and usefulness to you, the reader and seeker. It is important always to remember the direct object of Christ's healing love: Wholeness in the Lord Jesus.

As we conclude, we cannot but see how rich, in spite of poverty, man is before a God who can only love and heal. To a God Who continues to shower upon the land the richness of His sacred blood, may we be ever grateful. May that precious blood heal us from all illness; may it free us from within ourselves. And if it be the road of Divine Providence that man must bear the effects of sin that flow from his broken humanity, may God's redeeming grace give man *spiritual insight*. The words and thoughts of Louis E. Bisch come into my thoughts, as recorded in *Leaves of Gold*:*

Illness knocks a lot of nonsense out of us; it induces humility, cuts us down to our own size. It enables us to throw a search light upon our inner selves and to discover how often we have rationalized our failures and our weaknesses, dodged vital issues and run skulkingly away. For only when the way straightens and the gate grows narrow, do some people discover their soul, their God, or their life work. . . . Even pain confers spiritual insight, a beauty of outlook, a philosophy of life, an understanding and forgiveness of humanity— in short, a quality of peace and serenity—that can scarcely be acquired by the "owner of pure horse flesh." Suffering is a cleansing fire that chars away much of the meanness, triviality and restlessness of so-called "health." Milton declared, "Who best can suffer, best can do." The proof is his *Paradise Lost* written after he was stricken blind.

* C. F. Lytle, ed. (Williamsport, Pa: Coslett Publishing Co., 1948), p. 14.

12

SOUND THE TRUMPET, PROCLAIM THE FAVORS OF THE LORD

HYMN TO PROVIDENCE

Shout for joy to Yahweh, all virtuous men,
praise comes well from the upright hearts;
give thanks to Yahweh on the lyre,
play to him on the ten-string harp;
sing a new song in his honor,
play with all your skill as you acclaim him!
The word of Yahweh is integrity itself,
all he does is done faithfully;
he loves virtue and justice,
Yahweh's love fills the earth. (Ps. 33)

Aleph	*I will bless Yahweh at all times,*
	his praise shall be on my lips continually:
Beth	*my soul glories in Yahweh,*
	let the humble hear and rejoice.
Ghimel	*Proclaim with me the greatness of Yahweh,*
	together let us extol his name.
Daleth	*I seek Yahweh, and he answers me*
	and frees me from all my fears. (Ps. 34)

. . . fill your minds with everything that is true, everything that is
noble, everything that is good and pure, everything that we love
and honor, and everything that can be thought virtuous or worthy
of praise. (Ph. 4:8)

A soul in union with God is always in springtime. A soul in springtime basking in the sunshine of God's grace will share a special
union with the Almighty. Such a soul will eventually need to proclaim to the world the causes and effects of this human and divine
interaction. Sometimes the task of unfolding these events is an arduous one; it almost seems futile to try to express them adequately
through the various forms of artistry (writing, painting, music, etc.).
One attempts to expose them as something new, even in spite of the
fact that others may have done so before, and with much more force
and artistic skill. Fortunately, however, bypassing defeatism, we see
that among the living there are those who come forth with bright
new inspirations—as new stars. And they are truly skilled in telling
their own, personal story of eventful and meaningful experiences.
From the inner being of their souls, they burn with the desire to
spring forth and witness to the Lord Jesus Christ and the wonderful
mercy and love He has bestowed upon them. In so doing, there is
the added hope that their story will muster other souls and possibly
even other generations to relish the goodnesses of the Lord.

To witness to the Lord is a beautiful personal experience, very intimate and sacred indeed. One's conscience is very sacred; nobody
should dare to intrude on those sacred precincts. Telling one's story
is most relieving, for it serves as a catharsis that not only ventilates
the inner soul's burden but also offers reparation to the hearer of the
Good News. As one is blessed by God in the Almighty's own personal dealing with the soul, so does one become a sharer in the life
and mission of the Church. The WORD of God has spoken, and
the soul has listened to that WORD with reverence and with accep-
tance/surrender, the very ultimate and most powerful element for
healing. Reinvigorated, renewed in righteousness, that soul reborn
now goes forth humbly and joyfully to proclaim that divine romance
confidently. In so doing, it fulfills a prophetic role by welcoming and
announcing the WORD of God. In reality, such a soul is a channel
of grace to an evangelizing mission to community.

The historical fact of the first Pentecost is a reality of discipleship well seen and experienced in the early Church. There is a

supreme task therein to discipleship. It is that which belongs to the mission of the Church. That supreme task is not revival, but preaching the gospel to *all people*. Whether their skin be black or yellow, red or white, it is the job of the disciple to reach them with the gospel. Next to that of love, Christ gave us but one great command: "Go you into the whole world and preach the gospel." The command is one of urgency. Soldiers in an army would be court-martialed if they treated their officers' orders in the cavalier fashion with which some of God's people treat this GREAT COMMAND-MENT.

The beauty of witnessing is that WE ARE CALLED, WE ARE CHOSEN, WE ARE LIFE TO ONE ANOTHER. Let each soul, in disclosing its story, sound the depths of a faithful and good God Who is Life and Truth. Let each soul breathe its sigh of relief as, in a spirit of gratitude, it enters deeply into the secret recesses of its own life. Let it muster forth from that personal experience a depth of sensitivity. Let it proclaim to all who would have ears to hear not a dim, far-off echo, not a feeble reflection, not even a fraction of that which God has done, but let there come forth the story of a human soul in struggle and in search being touched by God unto a new life, unto a new intellectual joy, unto purified affections, unto a new restful state of ecstatic delight where the Almighty is seen and recognized to be what He is: "THE GOD WHO HEALS."

When God heals a soul, He prepares that soul for witnessing. Jesus offers Himself in healing not only as redemption and liberation but also as the transformation of a soul's life as He has touched that soul, as He has influenced that being, as He has renewed and regenerated that person into a refreshing actual grace, a refreshing baptism of the spirit. Conversion is a personal experience. Its story is precious. By whatever paths the converts may come, all those paths seek eventually the utterance of that journey to restoration and health. He who is converted becomes a disciple. At first his discipleship is difficult, because the convert must witness the reality of his own personal accumulated varieties of living as they may have been quite contrary to the Christian path of Jesus. He may feel uncomfortable at having to expound those participations which he surrendered to the grace of Jesus. He may have to face an insecure world, one apparently not needing God or His supernatural. But in His search for souls God has many avenues to bring us to our knees.

The glory of discipleship is that as one surrenders one's right to himself through the salvation message, he begins afresh to live the substantial love of God without sham.

A true call to witnessing comes as mysteriously as being born again, being born afresh in God's grace: It profoundly changes everything. Discipleship which produces witnessing requires that one keep himself or herself in the love of God as St. Jude admonishes the early Christian converts. (Jude 21) When God sends a special blessing, such as healing, upon a human being, the Almighty is really carrying on His constant interest and work, namely, sanctifying an individual. In so doing, the Almighty is raising that individual to a very lofty plateau of freedom.

When a soul is saved by God, that individual soul recognizes that his personal life is no longer his but is meant for Jesus, his Saviour and Lord. In religious circles, today more than ever before, we hear much talk about decisions for many causes, about decisions for Jesus Christ. Our determination to be Christians seems to warrant such. The fact remains that God has chosen; we did not choose by being taken up into conscious agreement with the Almighty. But in His calling us we were brought into a conscious knowledge of our nothingness and of our ignorance of what God is aiming at in selecting us. God's ways are so different from ours!

The simplicity of real faith in God is to see how peacefully we continue to follow in the path God unfolds day by day to us—regardless of how his providence gets more and more vague as we travel on. At times we may have our own particular notions about God's divine purpose concerning our work or where it is we must go. But in the final analysis, each soul is mysteriously being directed by God with special orders and to a special witnessing.

When one witnesses about God, one is witnessing the presence of God experienced in his or her life. This is the effect of what is termed in charismatic circles the "Baptism of the Spirit." That Baptism of the Holy Spirit is nothing more—*nothing more*—than God's actual grace as an internal religious experience, or a prayer sensitivity to God's presence. The person receiving this actual blessing is receiving an individual experience of the risen Christ in a far more impressive way than ever before in his life. It is this grace that causes him to go forth and to share his encounter with the Almighty. He releases all that has rested dormantly within from the very first days

of his own water baptism and confirmation. The power of the Holy
Spirit draws this individual into more deeply meaningful moments
of devotional life, more substantial prayer, more fervent and more
regular reception of the sacramental life of the Church, a greater
sensitivity to the avoidance of evil and the doing of good.

When one witnesses externally to one's internal regeneration, one
does so in a spirit of lively faith. This spirit is not one of intelligence
and reason, but of a life that has been sincerely sensitized by the
"awareness of knowing Jesus," Who now in turn wishes to use this
individual to proclaim to a befogged society the works and wonders
of a good God.

And so in the following pages you will be meeting and you
will be journeying through the inner recesses of real persons who
want to tell their story of their encounter with the Lord Jesus. These
are the stories of real people with real problems and situations, people like you and me who struggle and strive, cry and laugh, suffer
and pray. They are friends, believers, lovers, travelers; courageous
and weak, rich and poor, affluent and not so affluent; some are pro-
fessionals, others are simple ordinary folk; these are people who are
fearful at one moment, bold in the next. Anger touches them, as
well as peace. Some are young and others are blessed with the
golden wisdom of the years, but in the final analysis, they are people
in search. In their own words, with their own descriptive manner,
they speak of their special world, which God has filled with wonderment and blessing, new dreams, new hopes, and new love. These
narrations are truly unique, special, and distinct, because each person disclosing the story is individually appreciated and loved by the
Creator of his or her life.

As you read these testimonies, these true episodes of God's
healing love, you can take this journey with these people in an attitude of a VOYAGE OF DISCOVERY. You will see how a Wise
God can take the tragedy of evil and pain, which are not His creation but man's making through sin, and through the healing touch
of Christ, the Wounded Healer, bring forth holistic health through
the rays of the Cross: reconciliation, righteousness, regeneration, and
rebirth. Enter with an open mind to appreciate what these people
appreciate. They were sick once, and so healing is very precious and
real to them. Try to grasp their very personal feelings with your feelings as if you were in their condition; perceive their thoughts with

your own thoughts and appreciate their ideas as ideas that have the
power to help you alter what is hard for you. Be genuinely sensitive
to their human emotions, which also bear the force of photo-
graphing your own responses to your own emotions. See some of
them with bodies that are racked with pain from accident and disease, crying as you also would cry when all other possible aids have
failed. Healing is precious to the sick. It offers hope. These people
are *really real*. You may see yourself in them. That's good! For you,
too, will then have been witnessed to by these individuals called to
tell their stories.

Our records are filled with thousands of reports of claimed
healings, many of which are substantiated by medical documen-
tation. The following testimonies provide a sample of the physical
healings that have occurred:

Jinx M. Gorr, Fitchburg, Massachusetts. Letter dated February 4,
1982.

In 1976, after having experienced a marked weight loss, severe
pain and an inability to swallow even water, I was told by my
physician that I had cancer of the larynx with less than three
months to live. I underwent surgery that involved the removal
of one-half of my voice box and was told that the result could
well be that I would be unable to speak.

On July 1st my sister-in-law invited me to attend a Healing
Service conducted by you [Father DiOrio] at St. Bernard's
Church, in Fitchburg, Mass. I willingly agreed to go with my
nephew who had been afflicted with an illness that confined him
to a wheelchair. Truly, I went to the service to pray for my
nephew's healing. During the service you called out that a
person was receiving a healing of cancer. Thinking my own
condition was hopeless, I did not respond. Soon afterward you
came down the aisle, stopped at my row and singled me out.
You identified me as the person you were calling, and I admitted to having cancer. You then touched my throat and
shoulder and prayed with me, and immediately I was slain in
the spirit. I felt something like electricity passing through my
body and my arm (that had been immovable) spontaneously

extended in an upward position. Throughout the entire service
I experienced a burning sensation and knew a peace that I had
never known. For the first time in my life I knew that the Lord
had reached out and touched me.

The following morning upon arising, I found that I could
speak and even sing! To my amazement, I had an energy that
allowed me to bake, clean house and do all the things that I
had been unable to do. I freely began to swallow and ate without choking. My weight began to increase and I knew a vitality
that had never been mine. My weekly check-ups became
monthly and then every six months. Now I receive yearly check-
ups and there has consistently been no evidence of a tumor.

I know that Jesus is my Healer and I thank and praise Him
every day for the health that is mine. But I am ever grateful to
you, Father, because I know that God used you as a channel of
my healing. You will always be a "Special Priest" to me because God drew me to Him through you. And this has to be the
greatest gift that God could ever give.

William E. Foster, Albany, New York. Letter from the boy's
mother dated January 19, 1981.

I attended a healing service on Saturday, 10/11/80, at St. Mar-
garet Mary's Church [Albany]. On that day you [Father
DiOrio] asked many times over and over again if a boy had
hurt his ear when swimming during the summer. My son was
not present that day, therefore I thought it must be someone
else in the church. I had written a note to be put in the basket
before you started services "for health in our family" among
other requests.

When after a long time no one was found in church with
an ear problem from swimming, I turned to the woman next to
me and said, "I wonder if Fr. DiOrio means Billy?"

The next day, after Sunday Mass, I mentioned it to Fr.
Malecki [pastor of the church], who said William was the boy
and to bring him to services that afternoon. . . . Billy, who was
19 years old, and I attended the services Sunday. We stayed the
3½ hours and Bill, who doesn't attend Sunday Mass regularly,

turned to me about 4 P.M. and said he was glad he had come to the services.

The following week we went to [my doctor's] office, as you can tell by reading his letter [below]. I am happy to share this news with you. May God bless you in your works.

From doctor's letter dated January 7, 1981.

I saw William Foster at my office on June 16, 1980 because of an ear problem. He was swimming and hit his ear accidentally when he fell into the water. There was bleeding from the ear and the patient had a cold.

On examination, there was a traumatic perforation of the left eardrum. The patient was placed on medication and returned on June 30th and October 20th for follow-up.

When last seen on October 20, 1980, the eardrum was healed.

Jon D. Reed, Buzzards Bay, Massachusetts. Letter from his wife, May Reed.

Jon collapsed on 7/14/76 with seizure. For 6 months we didn't know for sure if it was a stroke or tumor. When the tumor was diagnosed surgery was advised.

On Jan. 24, 1977, a malignant tumor the size of a small lemon was removed, but the surgeon couldn't get it all because some of it was in the nerve tracts of the brain's motor center. He told me that Jon had a maximum of two years to live. My reply was "Dear Lord, if that's your will I'll accept it and make it the best two years of my life." . . . Jon was hospitalized for 2 months during which time he had 6 weeks of radiation therapy. Jon had 2 good months, but by June 1977 the tumor had completely regrown. Jon was paralyzed on the left side, he was becoming very dull mentally, and his time was reduced to 6 months.

He converted to Catholicism in May around the time our middle son made his First Communion. Jon received the Sacrament of the sick and became Catholic. Despite our grief and suffering during this time (Jon was only 40, our boys were 11 and 7 and our daughter 5), Jon always thought about me and was totally unselfish.

A member of Fr. DiOrio's ministry suggested we go to the Thursday service August 11, 1977—our 15th anniversary. . . . We went with the intention of thanking God for our 15 beautiful years of marriage. . . . That evening Fr. DiOrio said there was word of knowledge. "There are going to be healings of many serious illnesses tonight and one will be a brain tumor." I didn't think it would be Jon, as there were 1500 people at the service. Within 2 weeks Jon's (1) timing returned to normal, (2) his coordination and reasoning became accurate, (3) his wit and sense of humor returned, (4) he began using power tools and (5) started driving. I knew something had happened. He couldn't tie his shoes the week before. I talked with doctors. Knowing his prognosis in medical terms, they felt a cat-scan was a waste of time and money but agreed to a brain scan. They were surprised to see that the tumor had stopped growing. . . .

We found out that there was going to be a service at St. Anthony's in Fitchburg on October 5th. We brought a woman who was very ill . . . and Jon was praying very hard for her healing and not thinking of himself. She received an instant healing and came with us to Carney Hospital on October 12th for a cat-scan. . . .

We had an appointment with the neurosurgeon on October 20th. He paced back and forth in his office and congratulated Jon. Jon said "what for?" He had not been in pain and wasn't really aware of his mental improvement so had nothing to compare with. Dr. Paul said, "I've seen cancers go into remission before, but I've never seen one disappear." He showed us the cat-scan in June 1977 where the entire cranial cavity was filled with tumorous mass and the midline of the brain was shifted to the left and then the one in Oct. 1977 where it was all gone except 10% and the midline of the brain was back to normal—right in the middle. Dr. Paul said, "You've completely baffled me. I'm not even going to predict what will happen to the other 10%." I said, "I do. When the Lord heals, He doesn't do a halfway job—He's going to go all the way."

We were both crying and praising God. We went to another

service on October 30, 1977. At one point during the service Fr. DiOrio was praying and received a word of knowledge. He said, "Jesus, walk into that brain, touch every nerve, cell and fiber, touch the motor center and all parts that control body functions." I felt Jesus' presence so strongly in Jon, was crying uncontrollably and knew he had been healed at that moment. Jesus walked into Jon's brain.

For 5 or 6 months Jon was gradually taken off some of the medication and went through a severe withdrawal. He felt lousy and didn't believe he had been healed. His medical background and scientific knowledge made it difficult for him to realize he had been healed because in medical terms his prognosis was dim. In March 1978 another cat-scan was done and it still showed 90% of the tumor gone. Then Jon believed, began proclaiming his healing, reached out to help others and began a beautiful spiritual growth. He also forgave people who had hurt him in his lifetime and received inner healing. In October 1978, the tumor was all gone. . . .

We were recently tried in that Jon had 3 seizures on February 21, 1981 after not having one for three years and three months. I (we) had faith that it didn't involve tumor growth. . . . We were told originally that Jon would always have a "seizure disorder" due to the scar tissue on the brain. His phenobarb medication was increased. A cat-scan was done on 2/24/81 and there was *no* tumor growth and no changes from three years ago. Before the cat-scan Jon said, "Every so often the Lord has to remind me to do things His way, not mine, and I must respect my limits." . . .

A healing is like a marriage in that you work at it daily. The physical healing is only the beginning, but the spiritual healings and growth from a healing are so beautiful. . . .

Gertrude L. Kucera, Danbury, Connecticut.

I am a convert to the Catholic faith since 1958. . . . Over the years my arthritis had become steadily worse—attacking my back, fingers, legs and arms. It seemed I was constantly in the doctor's office for shots to calm the pain. My body could not tolerate medication—only aspirin—and some days I could hardly walk at all. My doctor had deep compassionate feeling for me. He has treated me since 1969 for one or another joint inflammation and felt he could not do much more for me. He had suggested 2 operations on my knees—the last one was to replace my knees with plastic and steel ones.

Last year [1980] Father DiOrio came to Danbury. I attended 3 of his healing services. Then in 1981 he came back to Danbury and I attended each morning service (Monday through Saturday). Each day I felt the presence of the Lord in my life. Each day I filled out the prayer slips and put them on the altar. I prayed for all my family and friends and the people at the services.

On Thursday morning I felt the strong sensation to pray for myself. I told God I wanted my legs healed for I felt I was being kept from witnessing and working for Him because of the way I had to drag myself around and the pain that seemed to never leave. I told God I would use my healing for His Glory and I would be His servant and witness. I felt great peace after that. . . . On the way to the parking lot that morning I could hardly walk. The pain was more than I could take. I prayed that if God gave me one more chance, I would claim my healing.

Friday morning (October 9, 1981) I again went to the Healing Services. I felt weary, cold, and in pain. I prayed that if it was not my time to be healed, that God would heal those poor sick people all around me. At least I could walk with my cane even if I was in pain. Father DiOrio was at the services that morning. Just seeing him filled me with peace. He carries the Spirit so strong and just to be near him makes me feel it too. I thank God for using him in such a beautiful way. Father spoke so softly and gently and was so full of love and compassion for all of us and he showed us the love he has for Jesus and the Blessed Mother of Jesus, Mary. It filled my spirit. I closed my eyes and praised God as Father moved out into the church, blessing and giving the word of knowledge to the sick. I heard him say "someone is being healed of arthritis today . . ." and I thought to myself "Praise God." I was afraid to believe it could be me. Suddenly I felt the Holy Water hit me and I let out a gasp. I opened my eyes and Father was standing in front of me.

He took my hands and I stood up and walked toward him crying. . . . He anointed me with oil and I was slain in the Spirit.

Father came back to me and asked what was wrong with my legs and I told him. He asked me to walk around and then said God had healed me and to put my cane on the altar. I began to praise God. I ran up the two steps to the altar, put my cane on the altar, and went back to my seat. After Mass I took my cane (upside down) back to my car—I walked WITHOUT PAIN. I have been walking without pain ever since. I can run, jump, squat, kneel, and do anything normal. I have not been able to do this for many years. . . .

I visited my doctor for my routine check-up. . . . He pulled, yanked, twisted, and punched my legs. Ordinarily when he attempted to do any of these things, I screamed with pain. This time I smiled and praised God over and over for I felt no pain. He made me walk. I showed him how I could squat on my knees and I went out into the hallway and ran up and down. He stood with a puzzled look on his face and cautioned me to slow down and not risk falling and hurting myself. I told him how I always knew God would heal me. I told him the miracle was that I could walk and had no pain and that as far as I was concerned, I am healed even if the bones are still messed up and out of shape. . . .

Each day I thank God for healing me. I thank God for using Father DiOrio as His instrument in healing.

Besides testimonies of physical healings, we have received many inspiring letters giving evidence of inner healings of a psychological or spiritual nature. Frequently we find that they are intertwined, and a person is blessed with both psychological and spiritual healing. These inner healings have dealt with fear, depression, memories, and of marriages and family relationships, alcoholism and drug addiction, and various mental illnesses.

The following testimony is from Louise Sutherland, a young woman who claims healing of schizophrenia and alcoholism:

In December of 1976 I was diagnosed an acute schizophrenic and from then on through last July [1978] I attempted suicide eight times. Six of these were by drug overdose, three of which resulted in such deep comas from which recovery was not expected. The seventh occasion was a self-inflicted stab wound and the eighth was a desperate attempt to jump off the Golden Gate Bridge in San Francisco. All of these were a result of what I now know as the most grievous sin against the Holy Spirit: despair.

In July of last year I found myself in Worcester. I had never heard of Father DiOrio except through NBC Nightly News telecasts. In any event, I found myself sitting in the church one morning at eight o'clock for an eleven o'clock service, wondering just what was going on. It was hot. I had just been released from a psychiatric institution, the kind of place where I had spent much time during the past two years. During the service people were praying and praising, going through what I considered to be the "antics" of charismatics at that time. Finally, at a quarter to three in the afternoon I just got up and said, "What the heck am I doing here? It's better to leave now." After getting outside to my car, I realized that I was boxed in the parking lot—it was a surprise to see how many people come to St. John's.

There were two options: I could sit in my car and sweat it out in the heat or I could go back inside and watch this very unusual priest do what he does. My decision was the latter. Standing in the rear of the church, I said to myself, "All right, Lord, if it is meant to be, I am going to do what this guy does." Coincidentally, I happened to be dressed in red and white that day, which are the colors of the ministry. Very discreetly I walked up to the area where this priest was then blessing and anointing people and witnessed what I later came to know was a deliverance. Two things flashed through my mind simultaneously. One was of total awe because if I never believed in the power of evil before, I did in that moment. The other was that I felt hot and wanted to get out of the church again.

Father finished praying over this individual and as he completed the prayer of deliverance I said to myself, "The only way I am going to get out of here is by being one less body for this priest to have to dodge." So I returned to the rear of the church and stood near the statue of the Sacred Heart, getting as far out of the way as possible. He was almost finished blessing and anointing people on that side of the church and was going over to the far side. Lo and behold, someone about five places away from me said, "Father, will you please bless me?" Well, he blessed that individual but didn't stop there. He went to the fourth person, then to the third, then to the second, and I thought, "Oh boy." After what seemed like hours but I am sure was only seconds Father blessed me in the same fashion as he did those other people—but he also anointed me. And vavoom! Down I went. When I got up I looked at the lady next to me and said, "Gee, it's really hot in here; I have never fainted before." . . .

Having been on such tremendous doses of anti-psychotic medication I had developed tardive dyskinesia (an odd kind of shaking), a very bizarre side effect of anti-psychotics—and one that is usually irreversible. It is generally manifested in people who have been on such drugs a long period of time, like nine or ten years, especially geriatric patients. Since I was a young person and had not been on medication that long, my suffering from all those symptoms was a bit out of the ordinary. . . . At five o'clock, while walking out, I began to shake like I have never shaken before. Riding home I was bearing down hard on the steering wheel arguing with myself, "This is absurd. I went there for peace of mind and I am worse off now going home than when I got there." Finally I arrived home and it was still unbearably hot. Not only was I physically drained, but more importantly I was emotionally drained and didn't know why. Knowing that Father DiOrio had another service that night, I decided to drive back but I lost my way. . . . I pulled the car over to a Merit gas station near St. John's and said, "Look, Lord, if you want me to get there, then get me there because I am going to try it once more and that is it."

Within minutes I was at St. John's. Once inside the church I sat in the rear because the service was well in progress and there were people hanging from the rafters. In fact, there was such a crowd of people there in need that I first stood for a while in the rear of the church and for the first time in over two years, I cried. Part of schizophrenia in my case was that I had not been able to cry, to release. So I then sat down and cried and cried. I

do not know what Father had been saying; the first time I
remember hearing him was at ten o'clock. He said, "Okay, we
are going to do blessings and anointings now." About five or six
priests were on the altar with him and he began to send these
priests throughout the church. So I said to the Lord, "If I am
here, God, I am going to get to this guy." Of course many,
many other people have the same notion in mind. I know now
that it is not necessary to be touched by Father. In that moment of need I guess I was being led that way. Anyhow, I
finally arrived at the front of the church and received the blessing of God through the hands of Father Ralph. I was slain
again then—and for a long time.

That whole incident last July was the very beginning of what
I later was to know as progressive healing. . . . The first and
last steps of healing that Father repeatedly emphasizes are forgiveness and surrender. All the events and things that had
brought on my own condition had their roots in my past. The
details are not important, only that they required forgiveness. . . .

In my own case I knew that it was not enough just to forgive
inside; I had to make the physical move of going to certain people with whom I had been associated and actually asking their
forgiveness. I did that. The day is still vivid in my mind. I was
involved in a lot of litigation with some people. Frankly, they
did not want to let me in the door. I finally convinced them I
wasn't there for anything other than to ask their forgiveness. . . . I walked out of there and I was broken. It was
the beginning right then and there in that moment of forgiveness when I had nothing left to do but what Father often
says is the last step—and that is to surrender. I could not even
walk, so to speak. I was moving forward but I did not know
what was propelling me. I had nothing left. . . . It became a
matter of giving my all to the Lord—which I did, verbally, as I
walked back to my car.

Afterwards I came to learn what it really means to be in
Christ, to be in love with Christ. I came to learn the very important distinction between brokenness and depression. That distinction is Jesus Christ. . . . I realized it was the Christ who
was the answer. I learned that I could rejoice in that suffering

because that suffering, as Father's teaching clarified, has given me perseverance. Perseverance has created character and character has created hope. That hope is Christ, my psychiatrist, and I am free. Praise Jesus!

Many persons have received spiritual healings in which they have experienced forgiveness, freedom from guilt, repentance, and conversion of the heart. Frequently when a person receives both a spiritual and a physical healing, he considers his spiritual healing to be of greater value because it has brought a new meaning to his life. One such person is *Sister Madeleine Joy*, of the Sisters of Providence of Holyoke, Massachusetts, who relates the story of her healing:

Six years ago I experienced the Lord through the healing of alcoholism. I had been addicted to alcohol for a relatively short period of time, one year. But it was a very long year and the most painful year of my life, for I was no stranger to the fear, loneliness, denial, degradation and guilt that is so well known to everyone who struggles with alcoholism.

Throughout the year I experienced two three-month periods of abstinence, each time to return to a drink and find myself quickly re-addicted. As I entered the last three months of my struggle of that year, I entered a very rapid progression into the chronic phase of alcoholism. And I reached out in desperation to one priest, one physician and to A.A. (Alcoholics Anonymous). I attended one A.A. meeting and at that one meeting listened to a gentleman tell of a car accident that he had and of the separation of his family . . . all the things from which the Lord had yet spared me. I considered myself still to be somewhat different.

Three weeks later, on December 16, 1975, I picked up what was to be my last drink from a bottle of vodka I had received from a family. I took one drink which led to a second drink and entered into an amnesia-like state known to the alcoholic as a "blackout." In this condition of forgetfulness I continued to drink until going into respiratory arrest.

That evening I was expected out with five couples that worked for me, but I did not meet their expectations. The next morning I awoke in what to me were familiar surroundings: an intensive care unit in which I had taught student nurses five years previous. Looking down on my chest I saw a respirator; looking up, I saw blood, intravenous equipment all around my bed, and oxygen. I knew the cause was alcohol. I was concerned about the pain that would be my family's that Christmas and was worried about what my community might say. Shortly, I felt a hand on my hand and looked up to see a Sister with whom I had once lived. I heard her say: "Madeleine, no matter what ever happens to you, we will always be friends." I remembered later that God had loved me even then.

A few moments later the doctor entered my room. He was an Episcopalian physician with whom I had had a working relationship and whom I had known as my own doctor for five years. He looked disturbed as he sat on the bed with my chart and I heard him say: "Sister, I entered the medical profession to ease pain and you entered the nursing profession to ease pain. We have worked together in the hospital for that purpose, but today I cannot ease pain. Last week a student died at the University of Massachusetts with an alcohol level in his bloodstream of .4 and I would like you to see yours."

As I looked at my chart I was awestruck to see the same number with two arrows pointing upward and two crosses above the arrows. The doctor said: "I want to say only one more thing. From now on the life you breathe within you is no longer your own, it is the life of Jesus Christ in you!" He left the room and I felt my concerns receding and a sense of quiet come over me as I had never experienced before. I knew before me the strongest presence of Jesus Christ that I had ever known and cried out to Him: "Jesus, save me! I'm sorry that I've wandered from You. Take my life and turn it in a different direction and I promise You that I will do whatever You ask of me."

Sometime later my community arrived, and in sincere love offered me the finest help that was available in this country at Beach Hill in New Hampshire, where an alcoholic priest was ready and willing to counsel me. . . .

After leaving Beach Hill I returned to my community in Holyoke and joined A.A. There I met the most loving group of people that I had ever known . . . people that taught me to live simply according to the Gospel. Only one day at a time. They taught me to get down on my knees in the morning and beg God to keep me sober for that day, to ask forgiveness for all of the yesterdays, not to bear the burden of the future and if I had offended anyone that day, to seek their forgiveness before the sunset.

One day I returned to my office in Pittsfield to clean it and upon arriving in the office became very frightened. Looking around, I wondered what must have transpired on that December 16th. Beginning to panic, I decided to return to Springfield and find my A.A. friends.

On entering the church where the A.A. meeting was being held that evening, I met a teacher and he said: "Sister, you look frightened." When I readily admitted my fear, he said: "My wife is waiting in the car so I have to leave but I do want to say, 'When you know fear, call the Lord!'" I did not go into that meeting. I went home. Going into our chapel I knelt beneath our crucifix and called aloud the Holy Name of Jesus. I felt my fear leave me and knew that He was healing me.

Some months later I returned to Beach Hill to find Father John to share with him the fifth step of the A.A. program . . . the fifth step is very similar to a general confession, but rather than dwelling on behavior it focuses more on the causes of behavior. . . .

Upon leaving Father at Beach Hill, I was driving home to Holyoke and saw a lake so pulled the car over. Overcome with my own weakness and aware of a deep desire within me to be alone with the Lord, I rested my head back on the seat of the car. Feeling an overwhelming urge to give myself again to the Lord, I extended my hands to Him and said: "Take the pride within me that has caused me to be so blind to my own weaknesses and so slow to forgive those of others. Take that pride that has caused me to have high expectations of others and to want my own way at any cost. Take the sloth within me that has caused me to procrastinate and the anger that has caused me to resent and to be so hesitant to forgive." And as I felt His peace fill my soul I knew He had forgiven me.

Four days later I met Father DiOrio and through the laying on of hands he began interceding for my healing. Immediately I knew a return of health to my arm that had been numb due to a prolonged time in respiratory arrest. A short while later he prayed for the restoration of severe memory loss. During the time of my alcoholism, I had been to Rome on a pilgrimage for the handicapped and had very little recall of that week. So two days after Father DiOrio prayed over me, I was going to New York with a priest with whom I had worked when we went to Rome. Addressing him from the back seat of the car, I said: "Father Bob, what is the name of the convent that we stayed in in Rome?" He inquired why I was asking and I told him that the name of Maria del Solo kept resounding in my memory. He said, "Madeleine, that is not the convent that we stayed in; it is the one next door!" I remembered the pizza that we had in Rome and Pope Paul extending his hands in blessing over the handicapped. God had totally restored my memory loss!

Through Father DiOrio the Lord has healed relationships in my life. He has healed past memories and He has healed me of unforgiveness that I had in my heart. He has healed me of a punctured eardrum and He continues to heal me each day as I receive Him in Communion in expectant faith. I tell Him over and over the words of Mary, "Be it done to me according to Your word. For my spirit rejoices in God my Saviour!"

13

MARY: MOTHER-INTERCESSOR

A great sign appeared in the sky,
a woman clothed with the sun, with
the moon under her feet, and on her
head a crown of twelve stars.
Because she was with child, she wailed
aloud in pain as she labored to give birth.

(Rv. 12:1–2, NAB)

"O Holy Virgin, in the midst of your glorious days do not forget the sadness of the world. Turn a look of kindness upon those who are in suffering, who are in the midst of difficulties, and who cease not to struggle against the misfortunes of this life. Have pity on those who love and are separated. Have pity on the loneliness of the heart. Have pity on the feebleness of my own faith and the faith of others who remain feeble in their brokenness, despair and emptiness. Have pity! Have pity on the objects of our tenderness, my tenderness. Have pity on all those who weep, on all those who pray, on all those who fear. Give each one of us—give me, give us, the hope of peace.

We ask this through the birth, death, resurrection and ascension of Christ. Amen."

It often has been said that a priest honors two mothers: his very own, physical mother, and his spiritual mother, Mary. The truth of the matter is that the priest has two mothers; and both mothers, the one in the flesh and the one in the spirit, have been given to him by God. The splendor of this relationship is that neither is a rivalry. In many Catholic Christian homes the physical mother would lay her child before the altar of God and at the same time implore the protection of God's own mother, Mary, upon her own little one. This very act was done by this author's own mother when, according to devotion as sanctioned by Roman Ritual, her child was offered in surrendering dedication to God and to the maternal protection of Mary at the same instant that the mother herself was ritually "churched" in the act of thanksgiving for the safe maternal delivery of both herself and her child. (Rom. Ritual) This act of dedication was made on August 19, 1930, at the Church of St. Bartholomew in Providence, R.I. More than many others, the earthly mother spoke and whispered many a secret prayer to the spiritual mother. This author's mother often asked God that someday—if it should be in God's Divine Providence—her son would save his soul and the souls of many others, if he would be permitted one day to bless, consecrate, and raise Host and Chalice. And so it has come to be: The mother of all mothers has become the mother of this priest. For twenty-five years, preceded by twelve years of seminary training and fourteen years of personal home environment, the spiritual mother, the mother of Jesus and the mother of God's children, has protected me from many a hardship. Grace given so copiously and generously requires verbalized gratitude. And so it is that this chapter, on Mary, mother of the Son of God, is written.

The purpose of this chapter is to profess openly that my life has been replete with this spiritual mother's love and mine for her. Mary holds that place of first lady in my life. As God has given her to me in a special way, so does He grace other souls with His mother's protective love, with her concern, with her intercessory prayer. She is there available to all who sincerely would call God "Father," Jesus "Saviour," and the Holy Spirit "Sanctifier."

We who are called as priests to live a special and distinctive form of life have also been given the actual graces of that sacrament. Mary is one of those.

The mother of Jesus is very precious to a priest. She is also highly loved and honored by Catholics who understand her determined role. And recently, many wonderful and inspiring books have been published by non-Catholics who have begun to review her presence and her role in God's divine plan. One meritorious literary presentation on Mary's favorite prayer, the rosary, was written by a Methodist minister, J. Neville Ward, and published in 1974 as a Doubleday Image Book under the title *Five for Sorrow Ten for Joy*.

To a priest, the mother of Jesus is very important. She is present with him in all the phases of his sacerdotal experiences. Through the love of this first lady, the priest is able to have deep insight, great respect, and a profounder love for all women who come to him. He sees in each one of them the beauty of this fair woman, be it in virtuous reality in present existence or in the potential of "being born afresh."

A priest's vocation was born from love, Christ. His vocation is therefore one of love. Because a priest cannot live without love, so he, in union with Mary, finds a greater love of the Holy Spirit through the intercession of her who was blessed with the fullness of that Spirit. Mary is constantly interceding for the priest. Through this very love in which he is compelled to live, he, like Mary, goes forth to generate souls for the kingdom of God. Like her who has become *the spiritual mother*, so the priest goes forth to become *the spiritual father* to all persons who would seek Word and Sacrament. With every sick visitation, as he carries the Blessed Sacrament, he relives with Mary her own scripturally recorded episode of bearing Christ within her womb as she made her journey to her cousin Elizabeth.

Mary is present to the priest especially in moments of weakness and other annoying failures. He trusts in her maternal concern, her maternal intercessory prayer before the throne of the Great High Priest. In those moments of healing, Mary helps him to uplift himself again to the standard of his vocation and to understand better the beautiful Church he is called to serve.

As Mary suffered the pangs of desolation when she had lost her Son, Jesus, for three days, so does she suffer the pains of her spiritual maternity when a priest might be slipping away. Mary and her weak spiritual son the priest suffer together. But as in the Temple when she found her Son, Jesus, she rejoiced, so too when she seeks her spiritual son the priest, finds him, and restrengthens him, she becomes Joy personified. Herein it is realized that through Mary's concern and care for the priest son, the Church of which she is the mother reveals itself more clearly as the priest's mission to all peoples. How well he realizes that he is ordained for souls! Through her own suffering, Mary teaches the priest that the wounds of the world are his to attend and to heal. He lives with her in life; and after his death, as he approaches the portals of heaven, he recognizes the welcoming embrace of his celestial mother, Mary, who had terrestrially accompanied him with faithfulness to the end of his pilgrimage and led him into the presence of God.

Many observers of my priestly life look upon my ecclesial mission of Healing-Evangelism with reverence and admiration. Inquisitively, and rightly so, they humanistically seek some sort of answer. Frequently, both by clerics and laymen, the question as to why God has chosen me and why God has blessed me is posed. I cannot answer that query, since I do not enjoy at my beck and call the extraordinary privilege of a "special messenger" of His Divine Providence. The answer lies in mystery. What I do know, and what I can respond, is that throughout the years of my whole life the Mother of God, Mary, was there! In each phase of my life's unfolding, this lovely lady, Mary, fulfilled her role both as my spiritual mother and as my celestial intercessor. This Blessed Lady was there nourishing, enriching, directing, guiding, and protecting.

Having a personal love for the Mother of God, having been the recipient of her maternal spiritual role, I hope that this chapter will not only be read but received and understood as one of the most important forces, *par excellence*, to my life and mission in the Church. This chapter also aspires to reveal in some succinct fashion how Mary being the mother of the Wounded Healer, Christ Crucified, is also by His intent the mother of wounded humanity. Being such, Mary in turn, through her maternal intercessory power of love and presence before the Holy Trinity, can seek to renew all things to God through her Healer Son, Jesus, who has gifted us His Holy Spirit.

It is also this author's hope that through this chapter many souls will come to know Mary and be led to her maternal heart. These pages are dedicated in a particular way to the pure, unsophisticated spirits, to those who desire to go to Jesus through Mary. To those who may not know her well because of time, circumstances, conditions, or because of some fear concerning her role, due to lack of profounder knowledge, may this chapter reveal her as God's created best.

It is a common axiom of psychology that before we can love people we must necessarily respect them. To respect people indicates that we like them for who they are and for what they represent. In Mary, prior to loving her, we respect who and what she is because of the fullness of God dwelling in her. In so responding, we express devotion. Devotion to Our Lady is an act of grandeur. In the lives of countless souls, devotion to Our Lady has mustered warmth and richness to man's service of God. Many souls have also experienced depth and beauty in their own cultural accomplishments. Any Marian veneration is associated always with Christ. With Him she forms sound structure and reliable economy for man's salvation.

Our Lady had a purpose, therefore, in God's divine creation of her. Everything in life is designed for a purpose. A thermometer is made for registering temperatures. A lawnmower is made to cut grass. But a mother's heart was meant to share the joys and sorrows of her children. So Our Blessed Lady not only brought the Incarnate Word into the world, but she actually and actively shared intimately in that very labor He came to accomplish: the healing and the redemption of mankind. Precisely because of this full implication of her relationship with God and mankind, Our Blessed Lady possesses a unique and exalted place in Christian life. The Christian spirit venerates her in dogma, liturgy, and general practice. Mary is the greatest external grace the human soul can encounter. The Church did not create Mary, nor did it make her important. It was God alone Who dreamed of her. It was God Himself Who transferred the blueprint of His mind into the reality of this humble Jewish maiden. In the very beginning of time, God promised that Mary would be the woman who would cooperate with Him in giving each one of us eternal life. In that garden of Eden, in the very presence of Adam and Eve, God said to Satan: "I will make you enemies of each other: you and the woman, your offspring and her offspring. It will crush your head and you will strike its heel." (Gn. 3:15) It was Mary with her seed, her Son, Jesus, who was to crush the head of

the deceiver and destroyer of the human race. Mary is God's
mother! Mary is our mother; Mary is our hope! Mary is the mother
of the Church, God's people.

A poet once wrote that the only happy man is the man closest to
God. All that has been given to us by the hand of God has been
granted only in so far as it is to lead us to God. But the loveliest and
finest of God's creations, which He Himself prepared and shared
with each and all of us, is THE MOTHER OF MOTHERS, Our
Lady. The greatest thing on earth is a mother. The very word
mother is significant of *life*. Mothers are the restorers of the home
and society. Pius XII used to state that the very destinies of the individual, of society, the Church, and the state are in the hands of
mothers. A mother is a child's visible guardian angel. Win a mother
and you win a family for Christ. Lose a mother and you lose a family for Christ.

The glory of Mary is involved in the Son-and-mother relationship.
All her privileges and blessings were given her for the sake of her
Son. Our Lady was immaculate, she was a virgin, she was taken into
heaven because she is the mother of Jesus. At that precise moment
when she said yes to the angel, she became the mother of the Word
Incarnate. She affirmed all that was involved in His life on earth as
part of hers. And so, His suffering, His death, His resurrection—all
these made her the spiritual mother of the world.

As Mary among all creatures held and will hold forever the first
place in the heart of Christ, so also Christ wishes that, next to our
love for Him and our worship of the Holy Trinity, His Blessed Lady
should receive our principal devotion. To honor Mary is to honor
Our Lord Himself. When we look at her life, the reality of the historical Jesus is introduced. If one ever wants to know the real qualities of a man, judge him not by his attitude to the world of com-
merce, nor by his outlook on business, nor even by his congenial
manners. Judge him, rather, by his attitude toward his mother. For
he will convey that same attitude to other women who come across
his path. When we look at Jesus as the Son of Mary, we perceive
the profound respect and obedience He surrendered to her, this creature of His Father's making. We penetrate His mind and His will,
and we see how very much He loved this woman Mary.

I feel it expedient to share with the reader very succinctly "essential reasons" why Our Blessed Lady holds a special place in my

life and in my ministry. To present her only as a devotion or as an object of piety without a substantial theological context would be, as some have trenchantly appraised it, a veritable monstrosity. Christianity with Mary in her rightful place will reveal itself as proper and sensible Christianity. And if this be true in the realm of doctrine, so it follows as veritable in devotion and cult. In the long run, Mary will be seen as the person *par excellence*, as the intercessor for mankind's healing.

Mary is the most charismatic of all creatures, because she, above everyone else, has received the fullness of the Holy Spirit. Certainly she is not a substitute for the Holy Spirit, nor do we attribute to her what belongs both to Jesus and to the Holy Spirit by absolute priority. She is sanctified "preeminently" in an incomparable way, as the humble maiden of Nazareth whom the Holy Spirit overshadowed in a uniquely charismatic and profound way. Moreover, Our Lady appears to us as a *real creature* privileged by the Spirit—as His most outstanding creation. For this reason, Our Blessed Lady can only be looked upon as under the light of the Holy Spirit. In so doing, we ourselves can see the Holy Spirit dwelling and working in a similar fashion within our own being.

Instead of looking upon Mary as an obstacle, we can look upon Mary, rather, as a way to visible unity, as a visible sign for healing the broken body, the Church. In truth, Mary will be fulfilling her role as a mother, nurturing and nursing her children. She will be seen as assisting in the healing of God's family. When Jesus was hanging on the cross and said to her that she should behold the disciple John, it was at that precise moment that she was giving birth to the members of the Church. Would it not, then, be most appropriate to recognize this mother as made by God for His Christ? Would it not be most beneficial to understand her as a mother of Jesus' family, the Church?

If we read the signs of the times, we can believe that all Christians will recognize the signs of unity as coming closer. Mary is the light of Christian illumination, as she is the star of ecumenism. Sometimes a star is hidden by clouds of darkness, clouds that are ominous, clouds of doubt or perplexity. But the star is there! For a star to be authentic, before it can be visibly recognized and trusted it must be understood in its essential components. It must be sound. It must be built upon truth. God is truth. He would not deceive.

God's Divine Providence has ushered in Christ by His Spirit through Mary.

The Vatican Council II (67, Dogmatic Constitution on the Church) devoted the entire eighth chapter to the Blessed Virgin Mary, Mother of God, in "The Mystery of Christ and the Church." It proclaimed that in Mary the Church joyfully contemplates, as in a spotless model, that which the Church herself wholly desires and aspires to be. It furthermore stated: "It is the first time, in fact, and saying it fills our souls with profound emotion, that an Ecumenical Council has presented such a vast synthesis of the Catholic doctrine regarding the place which the Blessed Mary occupies in the mystery of Christ and of the Church."

The Council was sensitive to other Christian views. John XXIII hoped to promote Christian unity, but he also knew that there existed differing Christian views about Mary. The Council spoke of Our Blessed Lady as "Mediatrix" (as strengthening and not lessening). It stressed Christ as the one essential Mediator.

In speaking of Mary, the Council used the biblical approach. It gave tremendous stress to the concept of "pilgrimage of faith." And the Council did not render any signs that Mary is separate from its treatment of the Church. When it discussed Our Lady, it accented the mystery of Mary in the larger mystery of Christ and His Church. The Council also stated that the practices and exercises of devotion toward the Mother of God should be that recommended by the teaching authority of the Church throughout the centuries. And it stated that these are to be esteemed. It cautioned theologians and preachers to be careful to refrain from exaggerations, and to respect the teaching of the Church as the dignity of the Mother of God.

The all-important fact is that Mary is inseparably united to her Son both as to His mission and in His message. Mary shared in the whole redemptive mystery of Christ. And for this reason she is inseparably united to His Church, of which she is the mother. Because she is the mother of all men—since Christ, Her Son, is the king of the entire universe—she is the mother of unity, who seeks by her intercession and love to bring all Christians together into one family of God.

To heal mankind, therefore, to save him, God could have chosen another plan of redemption altogether different from the one He chose. He could have sent His Divine Redeemer in the fullness of manhood, as was the case with Adam, the first man. But God in His infinite wisdom saw fit to have the Saviour of mankind be born of a virgin mother, whose free consent should be necessary before the incarnation could be accomplished. The Fathers of the Church present various reasons for the adoption of this plan by God; some of them are based on the fact that God is all-powerful, still others accent His greatness, goodness, and love. But the reasons commonly presented by all are those based on God's wisdom.

a) It is in conformity with the infinite wisdom of God that He should accomplish the work of redemption and vanquish Satan by the same means and instrument with which the latter had brought about our ruin. Satan had vanquished the first man through the first woman. Hence it was appropriate that the Divine Wisdom should also bring about our redemption by the instrumentality of a woman.

b) By being born of a woman, the Redeemer raised the whole human nature to a high honor in which both sexes share. And so the redemption of both is thus indicated.

c) As the dogma of the Incarnation is the foundation of the whole Christian religion, it behooved Divine Wisdom to accomplish the mystery of the Incarnation in a manner that would counteract the erroneous explanations of the mysteries deduced by other Christian beliefs as well as unbelievers. These opposing thoughts are refuted by the fact that the Redeemer has become flesh of our flesh, bone of our bone, truly born of a human mother and therefore truly man, one Divine Person with both the human nature and the Divine. If Christ had come in full manhood, as was the case of Adam, He would not have contracted such an intimate union with our nature. He would have been similar to us but would have remained a stranger to our blood and race. And for that reason, we could not consider ourselves properly His brethren and coheirs.

Through the mystery of the Incarnation, God sent us His Son to be the Healer of our wounds. Mary was the instrument of God to bring this event into reality. Satan used Eve to influence Adam unto sin. The parallelism between Eve and Mary is very interesting. The early Fathers of the Church insist much on the idea that as Eve

cooperated in the fall of humanity, so Mary cooperated in human-
ity's salvation. Holy Scripture clearly confirms the contrast between
Jesus Christ, the second Adam, and the first Adam. Thus we read in
Romans 5:12–19:

> Well then, sin entered the world through one man, and through sin
> death, and thus death has spread through the whole human race be-
> cause everyone has sinned. Sin existed in the world long before the
> Law was given. There was no law and so no one could be accused of
> the sin of "lawbreaking," yet death reigned over all from Adam to
> Moses, even though their sin, unlike that of Adam, was not a matter
> of breaking a law.
>
> Adam prefigured the One to come, but the gift itself considerably
> outweighed the fall. If it is certain that through one man's fall so
> many died, it is even more certain that divine grace, coming through
> the one man, Jesus Christ, came to so many as an abundant free
> gift. The results of the gift also outweigh the results of one man's
> sin: for after one single fall came judgment with a verdict of con-
> demnation, now after many falls comes grace with its verdict of ac-
> quittal. If it is certain that death reigned over everyone as the conse-
> quence of one man's fall, it is even more certain that one man, Jesus
> Christ, will cause everyone to reign in life who receives the free gift
> that he does not deserve, of being made righteous. Again, as one
> man's fall brought condemnation on everyone, so the good act of
> one man brings everyone life and makes them justified. As by one
> man's disobedience many were made sinners, so by one man's obedi-
> ence many will be made righteous.

And in the First Letter to the Corinthians (15:21), we read:

> Death came through one man and in the same way the resurrection
> of the dead has come through one man.

Scripture therefore clearly affirms that Christ is the new Adam.
Now, as the first Adam was not alone in the work of our ruin, so
the second Adam was not alone in the work of our redemption. Although the ruin of the whole human race was caused formally by
Adam as the head of mankind, yet Eve contributed to that ruin, as
we know from Scripture. She first listened to the temptation of
pride: ". . . you will be like gods. . . ." (Gn. 3:5) She was the
first to question the rights of the Creator: "Why has God commanded?" She was the one who offered the forbidden fruit to
Adam, after she herself had eaten of it. She thus cooperated in the

sin of Adam not as an irresponsible instrument but as a truly guilty party. Likewise, in the work of restoration of the human race, although Christ is actually and fully accomplishing our redemption, Mary is truly playing the part of a responsible agent of healing and restoration. She does this by her free and gracious consent to the incarnation of the Divine Word and by her active part in the sufferings of Christ.

It is worthwhile to point out this parallelism between the first Eve and the second:

a) As Eve prepares the way to sin, so Mary prepares the way to healing and restoration.

b) To the pride of Eve, Mary opposes the most loving humility, responding to the angel Gabriel: "I am the handmaid of the Lord." (Lk. 1:38)

c) The similarity that appears in the narration of the fall and the narration of the annunciation is a parallelism of contrasts. Thus the serpent, the bad angel, is contrasted with the good angel, the disobedience of Eve with the obedience of Mary.

d) Eve is cursed in her generation: "I will multiply your pains in childbearing." (Gn. 3:16) On the other hand, Mary is blessed in hers: "The Lord is with you." (Lk. 1:29)

e) The first narrative, that of destruction, opens the Old Testament; the second, that of healing and restoration, opens the New Testament. Mary gives us the fruit of life, whereas Eve gave us death.

Theologians have raised the question whether God himself clearly and explicitly indicated this antithesis between Mary and Eve in the passage of Genesis (3:14) where He inflicts punishment on Satan in the form of a serpent: "Then Yahweh God said to the serpent, 'Because you have done this, be accursed beyond all cattle, all wild beasts. You shall crawl on your belly and eat dust every day of your life.'" Then, in Genesis 3:15, God continues the condemnation of enmities between the seed of Satan and the seed of Mary who will crush the author of evil. This very text reveals the plan of divine healing and restoration; and it indicates that the woman in question is no other than Mary. Many theologians answer in the affirmative and declare that Mary not implicitly appears as the contrast in the narrative of the fall and of the annunciation but that God clearly and explicitly reveals this fact in these words of Genesis. Other theologians, however, though fully granting that this passage clearly indicates the prophecy of the future reparation, healing, and restoration for the sin of Adam, deny that there is definite indication concerning the manner of this redemption and the agent who is to accomplish it. They hold that it is only in the subsequent prophecies and especially in the narratives of the annunciation that "seed of the woman" meant Our Blessed Lord and that therefore the woman in question is no other than the Blessed Virgin Mary. We may conclude that in the light of the combined facts of the fall and reparation, Mary, the new Eve, enters into the very essence of Christianity, and that we must actually consider her as having a necessary share in the plan of the world's healing and restoration. We must, moreover, consider her role in the plan of the Wounded Healer, Christ the Redeemer.

In Mary, one can find all that the prophets of old foretold: through her all *expectancy* was fulfilled. *That expectancy* dwelled in her soul.

Mary was not the Mother of God by one isolated instance: Bethlehem. No! She is and remains MOTHER OF GOD— THEOTOKOS (θεότοκος, i.e. God-bearer, mother of the Incarnate Word). The fact of this motherhood is a reality fulfilled in time. Likewise, this even gives each one of us *the expectant faith, the expectant hope that somebody did become the Mother of God.*

This true story of God becoming man that man might become God, by choosing to become born of a virgin mother, appears paradoxical regardless of how beautiful the narration is or how relevant the truth it contains. By the mere fact of Mary's existence, there is signified that Christ, who became God and man, *had a mother.*

There is an old story that reveals that it would be enough for the Church, for God's people, to love her by thinking of her relationship to her Son; and from this reflection we draw theological conclusions. *Nothing more* would be needed for further contemplation than the factual truth that she is the mother of a Son called Jesus Christ, Our Lord and Saviour!

Dom Marmion, an Irish abbot of Belgian descent, tells the story about an old Irish woman who was always speaking about Mary. One day somebody was upset by that and said to her:

"You are speaking all the time about Mary. But she is a mother just like your mother, just like my mother."

The old lady looked at her friend and said, " 'Tis true indeed. She is a mother like your mother and like my mother. Ah, but the truth o' the matter is that *the sons are so different!"*

What a great consolation it is for us to know that Our Blessed Lady is ours as mother and as queen. From heaven's portals she continues to intercede for all of us. Even from her throne covered with glory, she always has her glance fixed on earth. She has placed her abode in us. Let us unite ourselves to Mary. Her glory does not separate her from us. WE ARE ALL AND ALWAYS IN NEED OF A MOTHER.

"Mother," cries a child in time of danger.

"Mother," sighs the adolescent whose heart begins to open to the most beautiful sentiments.

"Mother," implores the lonely orphan, because he lacks the most tender and sincerest understanding.

"Mother," calls a youth who, in the eruption of the most powerful affections, desires to have beside his heart a whole heart.

"Mother," invokes a prisoner who, far away from his mother, longs for her presence.

"Mother," cries the adult who has learned that everything that his mother taught him contains the wisdom of life.

"Mother," call the old man and the old woman who, on their deathbeds, seek the presence of her who cradled them at birth.

Mother! It is the most beautiful word. It is the only one that amply satisfies and indicates love, generosity, always ready to give of oneself in unreserved sacrifice. It radiates great and indomitable love that never feels rancor for any offense received. Truly there is nothing upon this earth that is more ineffable, immense, and indomitable than a mother's love; nothing more tender, feminine, and strong; nothing more touching and moving, nothing more capable of healing our wounds, than the love of a mother.

Let Our Blessed Mother heal us with her Divine Son. She is God's gift to us. Mary is the mother of the body of Christ, the Church. In being so, she helps to rebuild it with the spirit of Christ.

Our Lady heals us as she inspires us to be like her, who is our model and our ideal. As we imitate her, there flows into our being the healing love of her Son, producing for us a better life of peace, prayer, simplicity, and faith. She understands human suffering and its mystery. Because Christ, her Son, is always the central theme of her heart, she will best disclose to us her depth knowledge of Him. Until the end of time, because God has so willed it, Mary will be the woman of all times, the mother of all men. She is the mother to those who love her Son; and she is the mother of those who do not. She is even the mother of those who have never heard of her Son. Mary is the great woman for all the world—all those who have gone before us, those who dwell in the various continents of Africa, Europe, Asia, America. She is the mother of the clergy, the religious, all denominations. God has meant her for all men and for every period of time. If there is anyone who might express hesitancy or doubt as to the validity of loving Mary, let him reflect for a moment and observe how much Jesus Christ loved His mother on earth and continues to manifest His love for her in the mission He has granted her.

The more, therefore, we venerate and love Mary, the more we will honor and love Jesus, and vice versa. With an increase of love of Jesus, there follows inevitably an increase of love for Mary.

Shall we not turn to her in this final moment through prayer? Shall we not give ourselves to her who was the greatest receptacle of the Holy Spirit? Shall we not turn to her who is God's solitary boast, the *prima donna* in the world's healing and restoration? Let us go to her who alone was blessed to wear the red rose of suffering, the white rose of purity, the golden rose of victory and glory over Satan and his afflictions upon mankind. Let us turn to her who in begetting Our Lord became the mother of you and me. As children at her knee, let us pray:

> O Holy Mother, how great you are! You have given to the world your Son, Jesus. In begetting Him, you became my mother. All who would have God as their Father must, then, have you as their mother. Therefore, dear Mother, on this day, as I read this chapter, as I recite this dedication, I accept you just as God meant you to be, my mother and the mother of the Church. I renew my baptismal promises, I proclaim your Son as my personal Lord and Saviour. I know I have sinned, but I repent and ask forgiveness.

O Mary, as a sign of your pleasure in what I am doing, pray for the healing of the whole world. Intercede for my parents, be they deceased or living. Pray for that living martyr of humanity, Pope John Paul II. Intercede for our government officials, for our priests and religious, for all leaders of religion who serve you in faith, hope, and love, with prayer, patience, and suffering. Implore God for our parishes, our youth, the old, and the sick. Give us zealous and holy vocations—men and women who will go forth into the world to change the world and not to be changed by it.

Grant that our men, young and old, may love you as did St. Joseph; and that they may be found more frequently at your shrines imploring your protection and guidance.

Let our women imitate more and more your modesty in dress and behavior. Let mothers by their love for you instill into the hearts of their little ones a deeper devotion for you.

Grant that our children will always come to you for protection and gather around you as Jesus did.

O Mother, you have been made by God to be our guiding light, our star of ecumenism. Help us to make the journey of discovery and to follow that star that leads to the revelation of Christ seeking to heal us into an authentic Christian family of visible unity.

In our daily lives give us the wisdom of the crib that leads to the strength of the cross.

O Mary, as a perfect model of all virtue, raise us, your children, to the heights of sanctity. As a mirror of justice, help us to see and correct our daily faults. Mother of God, we are yours in time and in eternity.

14

LOVE HAS A MESSAGE

My dear people,
let us love one another
since love comes from God
and everyone who loves is begotten by God and knows God.
Anyone who fails to love can never have known God,
because God is love.
God's love for us was revealed
when God sent into the world his only Son
so that we could have life through him;
this is the love I mean:
not our love for God,
but God's love for us when he sent his Son
to be the sacrifice that takes our sins away. (1 Jn. 4:7–10)

If there were not some emptiness in our heart, would we ever
need God to fill it?

ARCHBISHOP FULTON J. SHEEN

LOVE IS A MIRROR:
There is no nobler experience in all of creation than that of man
loving his Creator, from Whose fingertips he has received life. There

is a double love in each of us. The first is a love that is self-realizing. It directs itself to our own benefit. The second love is that which effaces itself and looks beyond itself to the good of another. The first love is both egocentric and self-assertive. Its searchings are possessive in attainment. Such makes us eat, drink, clothe ourselves, enjoy entertainment, and even toil only with the intention to sustain our life. The other love focuses beyond itself and energizes one's ideals, purposes, and strivings. It is self-sacrificial. It does not possess but is possessed. It seeks not to own but to be owned. Its quest is not to voyage in search of treasures, but to open and share the treasures of itself. The first takes food and water that it may live, the other shares and even gives up the water and food that a neighbor may live. The first attends to his own bodily wounds, while the second heals the wounds of other men. It is characteristic of holy men that even while suffering themselves, they do not abate their concern for the needs of others.

Persons desire to be lifted up to the experience of love, and to be accepted by another human being. One can never hurt anyone when one loves him. One hurts another only when one rejects him. Mother Teresa of Calcutta is recorded as having said that the biggest disease today is not leprosy or tuberculosis but, rather, the feeling of being rejected and unwanted, uncared for, and deserted by everybody. There are two things that, once having been given, should never be taken back: one is our breath and the other is love. How many marriages are entered into in which love is pledged in ecstasy and then, after the character of marriage softens through its own crucible, love surrendered is now rescinded, becoming the carbon monoxide of the fleeting soul. The selfish person loves neither himself nor others.

The power of love presupposes its capacity to vulnerability. Vulnerability among human beings is indicative of people encountering one another. When God allows two people to meet, He grants them the opportunity to endow each other with their own presence, symbolizing Himself, Whom they both hold within. The interest and the concern they bear for each other even to the point of vulnerability is in truth He as their gift to each other. Transcending the human bonds of friendship, intimacy, and love, it is He Who is their bond of unity. In this encounter of love, God allows us to discover "the real" in our lover; and in the revelation of what is "real," each lover becomes increasingly vulnerable to the other. This love of that special person is a voyage of "inscape" or a journey within. It allows us to penetrate beneath the apparent externals: the eyes of the other, the alertness, their being alive, their responsiveness, and their fullness of promise. May God grant to each one of us as we read these pages and reflect upon them that we never superficially experience our loved one. The one we love passes by just once.

No pen would ever be put to paper were there not some expectation of good to come from it. May my words, therefore, transcribe themselves to print accenting strongly that true love strives to preserve and to promote the loved one as another *person*, not as another *self*. Neither does it render itself as a means of gratification— definitely not a tendency to "absorb" another's individuality for sheer selfishness. The test for those experiencing friendship, intimacy, and love is found in the question: Am I ready to bring about the happiness of the other person, even at the cost of a sacrifice to myself?"

Love is very complex, and so are the elements that it comprises. Love requires total demands. It is never easy to give oneself to another, not even to God. Because too few realize the cost of love—a total giving of oneself to the other—selfishness gets the upper hand. Because love is a total giving of oneself to the other, entering even into the wounds of the other, so therefore love is perceived as vulnerable. The pelican, it is said, actually pierces itself in order to nourish and give life to its young. So, too, Christ hanging upon the cross allows Himself to be pierced that the wounds of human disunity might be nourished by His own Precious Blood. Alone we are two separate individuals trying to survive. Together we are strength guiding one another unto the revelation of truth, maturing as we go into a world of dedicated love.

Men and women are made brothers and sisters through many ways: some by blood, but still more by sharing the same human experiences. Whenever life's circumstances allow us to laugh or to share the passion of fear together, we form bonds that help us to recognize each other as members of the same family. It is very difficult to look at another man as a stranger, once he has revealed his humanity to us. Strangely enough, one of the experiences that draw men together in understanding is the loneliness they feel when they are separated from one another. Separation is a strand woven into all human experience from love to hatred, from birth to death. No man escapes it. No man can solve the problem by himself, and no man who has ever been lonely can fail to be touched by loneliness in another.

When hearts are broken through separation, tears generally are the outlet. It is healthy to cry. It serves as a release from the inner prison of isolated sorrow. Tears say a lot, but sometimes they are hard to understand. We can weep for joy, as we can weep for sorrow. Tears have a language of their own. With each drop that flows from tear-reddened eyes, there is the adjacent mustering of anguish from the heart of him whose wounds bleed for the healing balm of another human touch. Does not healing consist in this: in the compassionate touch of another human being? As each tear flows from a wounded heart, so it is indicative that each person undergoes a distinctively meaningful pain.

It is a hard thing to cry, but it is not a bad thing. What is tragic is to cry *alone*, because this means we have built walls around our lives, walls so high and steep that nobody else can see over them. Our tears tell us that we are alive. Without tears, nothing can grow. Our tears redeem us when they reveal us clearly to another. Before another, we are unshielded from the consequences and the risks that are involved in being human. As human wounded healers, we should resolve that nobody who wanders the trails of lonely darkened forests, groping and searching as wounded seekers, should ever have to cry alone.

True love makes it possible for one to accept the limitations of the beloved. Genuine love is the most effective creator and promoter of human existence. When one loves another, he enters into that person's very wounds to nurse him with his own strength. Wounds that touch wounds are merged as life-giving transfusions. When wounds touch wounds, the grafting of another presence brings forth a new beauty. When one offers healing love to another, such a one influences that person to love himself. He helps him to accept himself as a whole person. He causes him to affirm himself and in so doing to complement that which God created in that person.

To love another is to desire his good. And at the very moment we have matured ourselves into loving him efficaciously, we have enriched that person. Antoine de Saint Exupéry is remembered as having once stated that love does not consist in gazing at each other as one perfect sunrise gazing at another; but it consists in looking outward together in the same direction. Henry Drummond himself compared love to a learning experience. In essence, he said that love is not a playground; it is a schoolroom. Life is full of opportunities for learning love with each day that passes, from sunrise to sunset. Life, for him, is not a holiday, but an education, and he concludes that the one eternal lesson for every man, woman, and child, young or old, rich or poor, sick or healthy, is how better he can love. Drummond finalizes that meditative analogy with a practical resolution that the constituents of this great character of love and learning are only to be built up by ceaseless practice.

Just as a flower opens its petals to a rising sun, so does a human heart open and respond to a hand of love. A kind, smiling face can be used by God to radiate the sunshine of healing to a cold and embittered heart. As it casts away sadness, it simultaneously disarms criticism, retaliation, and outright hatred. To love means to live for the sake of the other. A selfish person is always a lonely person. Real love is full understanding. It knows its own limitations as well as its own possibilities of error. It can sin as well as bring forth the blossoming of virtue. Interpersonal relationships nourished by genuine love are a badge by which a dissipated world is made to recognize the true disciple of Christ.

Each one of us has within his being a great deal more kindness and love than is ever spoken. Have we not shown expressions of kindness and love to many persons we have met? There are incidents that compose major chapters in our lives of which we scarcely spoke to persons whom we met; yet because we loved them in that particular moment, they felt honored and experienced healing love. How many persons we have met along the streets of our busy world! How often we sit with many a person in churches or theaters, with whom—though we may have remained silent—we rejoiced by some insignificant gesture of warmth. The effect of such an indulgence of human affection was certainly a sense of cordial exhilaration. From that highest degree of concerned love to its lowest degree is produced the sweetness of life.

True love for another, in the most significant sense, aids another human to grow. This growth allows self-actualization. The intrinsic beauty of such a dynamic exchange is that as we care for another, as we serve him through our own concern, spontaneously, without conscious realization, we find meaning in our own existence. No matter how love may be dissected, in the final analysis we realize that love is objectively the ability to establish healthy, meaningful relationships with other humans. Being satisfied, we find that our existence on earth unfolds itself as a successful life.

LOVE HAS NO BOUNDARIES! The greatest love story in all the world is God's love for us. There are thousands of people who have burdens to be lifted and scars to be attended to. Problems are abundant and they need to be solved. The world of pain needs lovers to nurse the anguished: to receive the emptiness that is part of human struggles. The love of God is a gospel to be lived out. This century, apparently more than any other period of history, is rent by scars. If in the language of romance there is no greater and deeper wound than the arrow of love, how much more bitter and painful is the sword that pierces the broken heart. Human love feels this sting. There is nothing more tragic than a broken heart. Interestingly enough, those who deal in interpersonal psychology recognize that a heart is broken not so much from pain as by the act of negation of that for which the heart was made: love. In order that one may understand this tragedy, let us consider a pain inflicted on you by one whom you love dearly. His bitter words are not what pain you but, rather, that he whom you love has done it.

There is nothing more traumatically shocking and conducive to a personality destruction than to experience that no one cares. Such an experience was undergone by little Mary Jane Elizabeth, whose home was the Abbott Orphanage, situated in a western state. She was eight years old, quite tiny for her age, and quite unwanted. So shy and so plain was she that you would call her unattractive. An alphabet of mannerism, unusual for an eight-year-old, made her feel "different." Other children shunned her. To her teachers, this "different" child was a problem. She had been transferred from two previous homes, and her present directors were seeking an excuse to transfer her again. The excuse was napping just around the corner. One afternoon, little Mary Jane Elizabeth walked through the main gate of the orphanage and hid a letter in the branches of a tree that cast its shadow over the entrance. For an eight-year-old, this feat was quite cleverly done. But someone had seen her. She had broken one of the strictest rules of the institute: absolutely no communication with the outside world without approval of the directors. The director and her assistant heaved the proverbial sigh of relief. Finally they had their excuse. Immediately, they hurried to the gate. There they saw a note only partially visible, peeking from between the branches of the tree. Eagerly and intently, the superioress, director of the orphanage, tore open the envelope. She read the child's large, clumsy scrawl. She did not smile. She spoke no word. With a facial mien of perplexity and embarrassment, she passed the note to her assistant. The silence of that moment was heavy, pensive, and more than a bit discomforting. The note read: "TO ANYONE WHO FINDS THIS—I LOVE YOU."

To me and to you, does not this story prove what we have firmly expressed concerning love, care, and thoughtfulness? We all need someone who cares about us, who accepts us for what we are and likes us in spite of all our shortcomings.

One cannot verbalize sufficiently about such excruciating and traumatic blows to life's existence. The following story reflects a pattern common among our wayward teenagers. We adults, having been sieved by the hard knocks of life, forget that perhaps the young have the same human need and care that we had needed and sought. A social worker tells this story:

A juvenile court referred a teenager's case to a Good Shepherd Home. Just seventeen, the teenager of our story wasn't really a bad girl—so the authorities said—but just a good girl that tried to cover the deep scars on her heart with rebellion, retaliation—a common reaction.

Her home life had been unhappy; her parents didn't even notice that she existed. She didn't belong; no one really wanted her.

After a few months in the Good Shepherd Home, the girl was granted a visit with her family. She chatted freely with the social worker who accompanied her for the visit. How eagerly she longed to see her mother again! How she was filled with happiness at the thought of meeting her again. Butterflies gurgled through her stomach with the excitement of the anticipated reunion.

They parked at the curb, walked to the front door with that bounce of anticipation, and pressed the bell. The mother answered the door. She didn't laugh or cry, neither did she open her arms. She was not surprised or happy. But she did manage to speak: "IT'S YOU . . . WELL, GET OUT. I NEVER WANT TO SEE YOU AGAIN."

It was a sad, silent ride back to the home. A human person had been rejected at a time when she needed response. A young heart had been stabbed, scarred, and twisted again. A young personality had been deprived of the interested care that makes it grow and develop. For this care, there is no substitute.

The girl must learn the hard lesson that *someone does care, even if those who really should, do not.* A young heart is like a delicate vase. It is so easy to smash into little pieces but almost impossible to glue together again.

These two incidents may appear to be isolated cases, but by no means are they. Rather, they are situations too frequently experienced today. In life someone must care. Someone must love. Thoughtfulness must find its expression. Everyone must emerge from his fearful, insecure prison and go forth to be wounded in order to heal the wounds of another. To be wounded does not necessarily indicate that we must surrender healthy morality and discipline, because all experiences cannot be undergone solely for the purpose of being able to say: I was there. Love, concern, and thoughtfulness will always, with God's grace, find their expression; SOMEONE MUST CARE.

To a certain extent, love makes a person what he is. Love draws out the best from individuals. Love helps the personality mature; moreover, love makes a person find his true self. Care, love, thoughtfulness are like the sunbeam and the raindrop that make the personality open its petals and flower into maturity. Care is the teacher that stimulates and encourages the raw potential of humanity. It is similar to a lighted match that warms the tinder so that it may in turn reach out, spread, and warm others. Care is truly a catchy virtue. It cannot help but multiply itself.

When one has a broken heart and cannot die, then one must suffer. Suffering by its nature must have an outlet, and this is usually in tears. Our Blessed Lord is recorded to have cried only twice, according to the Scripture narratives—once at the death of His friend Lazarus; the other, when He looked down upon the city of Jerusalem, the city on which He had lavished so many divine gifts, the city whose sick He had cured, whose blind He had made to see, whose lame He had made to walk and run again. With Lazarus, the Scriptures tell us, He sighed and moaned, and because He loved him, He had compassion. Looking up to heaven and then into the tomb of His dead friend, He shouted with intense deliberateness, "Lazarus, here! Come out!" The dead man came out, his feet and hands bound with bands of stuff and a cloth around his face. Jesus said to them. "Unbind him, let him go free." (Jn. 11:43–44) How often Jesus showed love and mercy to the people of Jerusalem, but they refused His goodness and rejected Him. Truly this was a bitter sort of suffering to His heart. If human love can feel this sting, how much more would and does the divine heart feel itself broken.

The world of pain seeks generous, compassionate souls. In those to whom love is not a stranger, the qualities of appreciation of pain, of cheerfulness, of a sense of the invisible, are constant companions. A tremendous difference is discerned between pity and compassion. Pain induces pity, which thereupon looks down on pain. Being aristocratic, it remains severed. Compassion, on the other hand, shares pain. It appropriates it as its own. It is more global. Its arms are outstretched like the arms of Christ on the Cross that was planted on Calvary's hill. Love blended with compassion becomes a journey of the heart. A human heart wounded in life has a propensity to recognize genuine love. Is love genuine in our lives? Are we real?

A little boy visiting Hollywood for the first time was intrigued by the thought that he was walking on a part of the land where "stars" actually lived. He was determined to meet some. One day while walking across Hollywood Boulevard he went looking for stars. As he looked and looked, he could see none that he knew. Suddenly seeing some nuns dressed in conventional habit walking by, he ran frantically, excitedly, and hopefully up to them and said: "Sisters, are you real or are you in the movies?"

Another story comes to mind of how love rejected leads to tragedy. There was once a wealthy man in New York City. Life had been good to him. He had many possessions. He had tasted all the types of pleasures that could be gained from the world and from people. And yet he was not happy, because true love for himself was never experienced. One day, he could not stand to live any longer. Life had no meaning, no purpose. He drove to the George Washington Bridge, a high bridge over the Hudson River, and parked his car at a side road near the entrance to the bridge. Walking to the center of the bridge at its highest point, overlooking the center of the Hudson River, he looked down—way, way down—to the river. With a life of emptiness behind him, with a future unknown and a moment of despair at hand, he determined that in a few moments he would enter that water and would finish everything on this earth. So he lit up his last cigarette, and as he was smoking and contemplating what he was about to do, his escape from reality that he could no longer support or sustain, a hobo came along. The hobo walked up to the man who was about to jump and said: "Hey, mister, do you have a dime for a cup of coffee?" The man who was about to commit suicide turned around and looked into the eyes of this bum from skid row. Such a ragged creature! The stench of his clothing urged fumigation. His speech was coarse. The wealthy but despairing man answered: "A dime, huh? I have much more than that. I'll tell you what I'll do. I'll give you more than a dime. He put his hand into his pocket and drew forth a wallet containing five-hundred-dollar bills. Looking into the face of the beggar and thrusting forth his arm holding the wallet, he exclaimed: "Here, take it all! Have a ball! Where I'm going, I won't need it." The hobo picked up the money and flipped through the five-hundred-dollar bills very rapidly. Somewhat perplexed, he questioningly addressed the generous donor: "Mister, why are you giving me all of this money? All I want is a dime. I feel more comfortable asking for a dime." The man replied in a dejected voice that almost indicated what he was planning to do: "I don't need it where I'm going." Suddenly the hobo realized what was going to happen. Excitedly he said: "You mean you're going to kill yourself? You are a coward! Here, take your money. I don't want a coward's money! And he threw the money at the man and began to run away. The rich man suddenly realized truth. Picking up the wallet containing the money, he rapidly paced after the hobo. What transpired in that one instant of their reunion is not clear. But anyone who saw them observed that after a few moments of talking they hugged each other in an embrace of compassionate, healing love. The story continues that because a poor man, a hobo, compassionately encouraged a rich man, a hopeless despondent, they were seen to walk away together not into oblivion but into the founding of a wealthy Texas oil company. How true it is that love is an efficacious attempt to help another: to seek his or her well-being. St. John of the Cross states: "Where there is no love, put love and you will find love."

When God allows two people to meet, He grants them the opportunity to endow each other not only with their own personal presence but also with the presence of Himself. Essentially, God is their gift to each other. He is their staunch bond of unity. For them, God becomes translated into human behavior as they grasp love as a warm and wonderful encounter with the essence of true living. Love is the core of all concerns. Love is the creative force for change. Love reinforces the importance of the individual. Love is not a path; it is a sharing. Love liberates a person from his enslavement, to true being. The tragedy of life is what dies inside of a man while he lives.

Many of us today are afraid to waste ourselves, our time, our energy, even our love. Many of us today seem to have forgotten that from the apparent impossible, great energies can be brought forth from those who have stifled such power. The gospel law exhorts us to give and it will be given to us, to spend and it will be returned more abundantly. To give of one's own resources, especially from one's own being, may appear to be a "waste" and a "futile pouring out." On the other hand, when we humans supernaturalize our "apparent waste," we actually are transforming a "seemingly human expenditure" into a "possible incredible grace." Theologically speaking, this is "grace working and embellishing man's nature." It is nothing more than an invisible vision receiving "birth" through a visible consumption. When we help another to beat anew with a heart of love, miracles take place. If we are unreservedly willing to waste time on others, we will enjoy the purpose of our living as we witness value springing forth in all its beauty. Yes, the impossible can be produced!

Everyone appreciates understanding, loving compassion. It is indicative of contact with others. Wherever Jesus went, there were crowds of people. No wonder. He spoke so comfortingly. He helped people in all their troubles, wherever they were: in the streets, along the docks, along the lakes, on grassy plains; He was always there helping people to be their best. How often Jesus saw the crowds enmeshed in all kinds of unhappiness! He felt sorry for them. He was moved with compassion for them. He saw that they were distressed and scattered, like sheep not having a shepherd. Jesus Himself gave them some good advice as He enriched the crowds with His messages. He told them so often not to be afraid but to trust in God and to be ready to suffer anything for God's sake. Not only did He exhort them and teach them, but He also in a practical way took good care of the crowds that followed Him. He not only healed their sick, but He also fed the people. They had journeyed so far from their homes just to see Him, just to touch Him, just to hear Him, just to love Him. Hunger and tiredness and sacrifice were no obstacle when they had come to know that this was no ordinary man. This Jesus of Nazareth was far more than just a Messiah, just an itinerant preacher, just a Divine Physician. To them He was what He came as: the Son of God. The people loved Him. Many times, they ran after Him over the countryside. They brought their little children to Him to feel the tenderness of His embrace, the touch of His hand, the blessing of His Father. He loved them so much that at times His heart would overflow with the sentiments of His inner spirit. His spirit verbalized His love by saying that some-day He would die for His people. To me, the compassion as per-sonified by Christ in the first person is indicated in these words: "I sympathize—I suffer with—I understand—I want to establish con-tact with a human being."

Today more than ever before, we are witnesses to an almost uni-versal urge, both on the part of individuals and of nations, to estab-lish contact with others. As each man gropes along life's trails, seek-ing to be embellished both within himself and for the betterment of the world, he must establish his contact with others through a more sympathetic, more meaningful, more realistic human touch. A per-son even in a crowd can remain quite alone from so-called "friends" unless he is willing to see them as they are and to welcome them into his life, to pick them up and give himself to them. A person should never be so inflated with himself that he forgets the other. Love and compassion in simple description is *thoughtfulness*.

There is an incident related in the life of President Abraham Lin-coln. Its simplicity bears an abundance of wealth about thought-fulness motivated by compassionate love. It deals with an old friend who arrived in Washington and called upon Lincoln at the White House. After a long, lively conversation, the President—accustomed to being plagued by office seekers and others asking favors—asked this friend what he could do for him. "Nothing," was the reply. "I just came here to tell you that I love you and believe in you." Much moved, Lincoln sprang to his feet, warmly clasped the man's hand and exclaimed: "You don't know how much good that does me! You are about the only man that has come here to see me that hasn't wanted something from me." To the day of his death, Lincoln remembered the simple thoughtfulness of a friend from far away, who wondered if Lincoln might be lonely in crowded Washington.

The signs of a great man will always be sympathy and compassionate love. It is a language all its own, a language that is understood by strangers and foreigners, even heard by the deaf and made clear to the blind. Thoughtful love always recognizes an opportunity to offer assistance, to express appreciation, as well as to enrich human sentiments with further hope and cheerfulness through strengthening words. Its joy that dwells within a person surrenders itself even to apparently insignificant creatures.

Another incident in the life of President Abe offers a related inspiration. On the day that General Grant's army made its final attack, President Lincoln sat in a small telegraph office scanning telegrams and studying a small chart. Suddenly three little kittens were running about the tiny office. Though burdened as he was with the care and worries of the nation at war with itself, Lincoln picked up the little kittens and put them on the table, saying: "Where is your mother?" The officer in charge answered: "The mother is dead." Lincoln went on: "Then she can't grieve for them as many a poor mother is grieving now for her sons who are falling in battle." Then, with his own handkerchief, the great President wiped the dirt from their eyes and again spoke: "That is all I can do for you, little friends. Colonel, get some fresh milk and don't let them starve. There is too much starvation these days."

Love is a journey of the heart. To love God, Who cries for union with us, is a journeying, a voyage of the heart. History has recorded many an adventurous voyager: thrilling in their search and overwhelmingly ecstatic in their discoveries. I can remember spending many a moment as a little boy near the old iron stove, keeping my body warm as I enriched my mind and imagination with the classical adventures of great discoveries: Robert Louis Stevenson's *Treasure Island*, the story of King Arthur's Knights of the Round Table, Jules Verne's *Around the World in Eighty Days*, Jack London's *Call of the Wild*, Mark Twain's *Huckleberry Finn* and *Tom Sawyer*. As enriching as these classics may have been in all their human beauty of narration, there is nothing more thrilling in journey adventure as the human heart in search of its God. It leads to the treasure of treasures: the discovery of God as Creator and end of our being.

Just as human voyages of discovery require sacrifice, so is it in the journeyings of the soul with God. Everyone who would love Jesus eventually must merge his wanderings and meanderings to the route of Calvary. Man's love is a vision unto the Cross. At Calvary's heights, new understandings are perceived with new values placed in balance. Strange indeed is this scene! There, on that cross, appeared a man apparently defeated: a man hated, a man condemned. And yet he who loves the Christ in His crucified love sees the paradox: In apparent defeat dwells victory; man's hate is met with Christ's love. Man's condemnation becomes Christ's forgiving love. The road of love along God's map is indeed a mysterious journey. It is God accompanying one on that journey Who takes the initial move to demonstrate His definition that He is love.

Encountering the love of God necessarily conveys our experience of Him to the love of neighbor. We must love both God and man. However, we never love another more than God, and human love must never go against Him.

Our encounters with man reveal to us the value of his humanity; but, at the same time, we proclaim with the psalmist of old that God has crowned him with honor and glory. Jesus, Who has loved us, has not only asked us to love another human being but also has established how to love another as He Himself loves each one of us. He demonstrates that human feeling is not enough—that actions are more concrete: "For I was hungry and you gave me food; I was thirsty and you gave me drink." (Mt. 25:35)

God's love is an intimate calling. One can almost picture Jesus with His arms always outstretched, whether upon the cross or along the walks where He permits man to accompany Him. He speaks of His heart in the Gospel of Matthew (11:29). His heart is a sign that He loves us. It is also a reminder that He wants us to love Him in return. He will always hold His people in His heart. In the First Letter of John, Chapter 3, verse 14, we are reminded that the man who does not love is among the living dead. Sister Josefa Menendez, in her exposition *The Way of Divine Love*, personifies Jesus pleading with the heart of man: "Look at My heart, study it, and from it you will learn love."

All of the great dogmas of our Christian faith should both shape themselves from and radiate themselves from the heart of Jesus and lead us back to it. To approach the Master, we should do so through

His heart. Precisely at His heart lies the Christ, Who is defenseless. He bears wounds through His vulnerability. As man himself remains vulnerable to those who wound his heart in life, so the heart of Jesus in all its sacredness remains vulnerable to receive and heal the wounds of humanity. His heart will forevermore be opened to hold all of His people. Because of His wounded love, Jesus saves your life from ruin. He crowns you with mercy and compassion. Let us worship Jesus, Whose heart was wounded for love of us. How little is known of the merciful heart of Jesus! He bore the burden of His love in silence until the moment came to share it. Then, one day as He was preaching, He suddenly gave Himself away as He disclosed His secret. "Learn from me for I am gentle and humble of heart."

Love by its very nature seeks union. God through love wanted total union between Himself and us. Men may hunger for God, but God thirsts for men. God's cry for men through His Son, Jesus, is a cry of thirst. It is the cry of a divine wounded heart craving for men, craving for little ones, for the hungry hearts, for the empty hearts, for those buried in the quagmire of sin. Many who have so much give so little, while a few who have so little give so much.

The thirst of God for men is also a cry. Could God in all His Divinity be more expressively human than this: to weep for men? Why did He weep? He did so because of all the goodness He had lavished upon men. They threw His goodness right back into His face. Rather than return love for love, man rejected His love. The Master freed each one of us from sin. At baptism, He gave each of us a new white garment as pure and simple as an angel's. He strengthened us in His love as He endowed us for His service, confirming us as soldiers in His army. But man, being engrossed in materialism and secularism, became ever more weak. He fell, like a wounded soldier, in the luster of sin.

The two greatest dramas of life are the soul in pursuit of God and God in pursuit of the soul. The first has less apparent urgency, because the soul that pursues God can do it leisurely. But when God pursues the soul, He proves a relentless Lover. He will never leave the soul alone until He has won it or been conclusively denied by it.

How often in life we make mistakes and rise again by the confession of our own guilt! We repeat time and time again that we love Him. And yet, we still fall. We repeat the old romance of sin and passion. We spoil our good resolutions. And the sacrament of re-

storal to God's grace remains only a memorable past consolation. Instead of the romance of divine love, penitent sinner loved and received by our Wounded Healer, we prefer to dance in the romance
of sin. But we forget that romance always carries a dagger in its scab-
bard. Often we receive Him in that holy union of love and agape.
We whisper to Him the secret stirrings of our loving heart. Enraptured in the moment of prayer, and in the experience of love surrendering to love, we promise that we will never walk as strangers again.
But as soon as we leave His presence, become distracted in an external rapture of worldly things, we walk away, not too far but distant
enough. It is always dark when one walks away from the light. Moments of prayer and intimacy must never be left as past isolations
satisfying an instant need. They should never be perfunctory. Whenever one walks with greater emphasis with things that are not divine,
one sooner or later blisters the cheeks of the Master with a venom-
ous betraying kiss of sin. Judas has had his day and received his reward. His behavior, however, perpetuates itself in man's incon-
sistencies.

This is why Jesus weeps. Yes, there is nothing in all the world so
tragic as a broken heart. He loved us so much and we apparently
hardly care. We rupture His heart, His sacred heart, through the
strain of wounded love. Such indeed is the tragedy of the BROKEN
HEART OF CHRIST.

My dear friends, what could appeal to one, more than a broken
heart? I ask you to perceive this fundamental thought of how God
loved us so much that He sent His only Son, Jesus, to love and heal
our wounds. He has borne care, love, thoughtfulness, and the
profoundest concern. But the paradox of love is that we who are
slaves to be loved deny the love that always waits for us. I think the
experience of most of us will verify this fact when we have deeply
wounded another. What draws us back to him is not so much the
wound itself but, rather, that that person continued to love us even
while his wounds were open, even while we were still unaware of his
love. "I love you, I forgive you, for you know not what you do." Like
a wounded soldier, scarred through battle, victorious in conflict,
Jesus shows His wounds to each of us—those five sacred precious
wounds: "Look at these hands—these feet—this heart pierced for
love of you." Do not resist His pleading love, which emanates as a
flame of sacred invitation. Do not leave Him there a forsaken Lover.

Listen to His pleas, which He made as He blessed the land of Palestine with His sacred footsteps and voice. Listen—come close to its resounding message as it rings from the cross. There He is, suffering, twisting, turning to and fro in anguish. Why? For you and me. Look! See His side! Pierced with that silver glittering spear thrust by the clumsy brutality of a boisterous soldier. Why? For love of you and me. Look on the ground beneath. There is John, the faithful priest, ever loyal to His Master—never distant from His gaze. Those who look into the face of Jesus as John did will always understand the profound throbbings of His heart. And there *she* kneels, that woman of renewed love. There she crouches with her face in her hands, with disheveled red hair covering the embarrassment of a past life—face and breast close to the ground from whence she came —tears mingling with His blood that falls to the sand. There she remains, ever faithful and loyal as the sinner of the moment who becomes the saint of the next.

Behold her who stands in valiancy—*Stabat mater juxta crucem:* "THERE SHE STOOD BESIDE THE CROSS"—not fainting, not drooling, but praying as she offers the sacrifice of the flesh and blood of her Son, Jesus. As she looks into those gaping wounds, as she sees those red rivers and torrents of rich blood flowing so rapidly and copiously to the ground, splashes of it even crimson her own face and garments. John and Mary of Magdala also sense the warmth of those crimson drops. The price of love is pain. But if the Cross of love and life indicates pain and anguish, it is the love of the Cross by Christ that changes its tragedy into the victory of divine love alchemizing the poverty and the leukemia of man's heart.

Who is he that can remain so insensitive to a love that cries with pain? Let not our hearts usher forth rejection and piercing. Let them not be like the cold steel spear that ran through that muscled heart with hatred and indifference. Oh, why, why must there be hearts who will love everything but Love—monetary gain, passion, flesh—who love without commitment? Why would man not believe that God loves him even in his hate? The power of healing love rests no longer upon the responsibility of God loving man. The power of healing love is similar to that of a bank that is filled with treasure to disburse. The power to be healed by the power of the Divine Healer, Who is love, rests upon the response of man to His God. God has done all He could to restore a divine romance. God has fulfilled the psychology of love supernaturalized by His grace. He spoke His Word; He sent His Word. His Word touched man as man can still touch Him.

You have asked me often how to be healed. The pages of these chapters have spoken to you of the power to heal. Return Him love for love by fulfilling the nature of love. All things considered, all books of all sorts written become only "little sparks" of description of what true healing love is: the love of a God rejected by man continuing to love him in his hate. His sanctifying grace dwelling in our souls resides constantly as long as we consciously reject and remove sin. Sin in all its forms is destructive of love. It is insanity. It is irrational behavior. It depersonalizes us into a "nothingness." God's love, however, as long as we still traverse the sands of earth, is creative. Out of the depths of our nothingness, God can make a new creation. And the response to this healing, compassionate love is to affirm decisively one's moving from sin into a constancy of union with God.

With all the love in my own human, priestly heart, a human heart that has tried to live in responsibility to God's calling, may I plead with you as God's visible voice: "Don't travel your life with a broken heart. . . ." The world today is a world of broken hearts. Oh, look to Him in all humility. Look at Him as He hangs upon that infamous beam of contradiction. Wooden beams clasped against each other—what a contradiction of God's will! His greatest suffering was not that nails should make His hands and feet red rivers of blood; not that thorns should encircle His divine brow with crimson drops of His redemptive blood; not that thirst should dry up His divine lips that preached the waters of everlasting life, not even that Mary's heart should be pierced by the seven swords of sorrow as proclaimed by Simeon; not that executioners ridiculed Him and diced for His garments in scorn—all this was bearable, tolerable. But what was unbearable was that they whom He loved should do it —that His blood should flow to a ground apparently more thirsty for His redemption than man; that Mary, His dearest possession, should be rejected and denied her maternal, caring hand; that Judas would pass on his blistering kiss of betrayal to cheeks that were divine; that He loved us so much and we hardly seemed to care. His greatest pain, epitomizing all previously described, is that He would be denied the possibility of holding His people in His heart.

As you reflect, then, on the divine love, you may be moved to surrender yourself to the Lord. But in doing so, you may be harassed and dismayed by thoughts of past moments that were sensitized by the ugliness of sin, by experiences that would be better forgotten than remembered. Discouragement may dissuade you. Perhaps in the conscious guilt of self-condemnation you feel unworthy to be embraced by His encircling, healing arms. If that be the case, may Christ's love, which is always positively flowing forth upon all mankind, continue its red rivers of purification and forgiveness. His love, brought to earth, both to you and to me, I believe can be best depicted in this story, with which I conclude:

It was many, many years ago. Before the doors of a magnificent church in Paris a poor beggar used daily to take up his stand. He had become a familiar sight there. The pious people who visited the church called him "Old Tom." By no other name was he known. His history seemed to be wrapped in secrecy. Sometimes, when the wind blew aside the greasy rags that covered him, a golden cross could be seen glittering on his breast. Some token—perhaps a dear mother's parting gift—so thought the kind givers as they generously responded to the beggar's appeal.

Old Tom, in his station near the church's door, soon found a fast friend. This was Father Pierre, a young priest who was accustomed to say mass at that church. Having abundant compassion for all whose lot it is to feel the weight of poverty and suffering, the young priest never passed the beggar without giving him a gift of money, accompanied by a kind smile and a cheery word. And the old man always thanked him with a countenance lifted up by gratitude and joy. He learned to love Father Pierre even as the young priest loved him even more.

One day, on coming out of the church, Father Pierre was about to make his accustomed offering when, to his surprise, he found Old Tom nowhere in sight. Several days passed and yet he did not appear. "What could be the matter?" he inquired. Old Tom, he was told, was sick and at home. Forthwith the priest asked the way to his dwelling place. In a poor quarter of the city in a dilapidated tenement, in a garret at its very top, he found Old Tom's room. "So this is the poor soul's home," murmured the priest as he rapped at the creaky door.

"Come in!" cried a feeble yet anxious voice. As the door squeaked open, there, upon a rude mattress at one end of the room, lay Old Tom. A glance that was complete in one sweep of vision sufficed to show the priest that the poor beggar would soon beg no more. He was rapidly nearing his end with a consuming sickness. The face of Old Tom, when he saw the unexpected visitor, was illuminated with a tremendous joy. "What, Father!" he exclaimed. "You? You come to see me?"

"Surely, and why not?" returned Father Pierre with a cheery smile. "Do you think I would desert an old friend who is in need, Tom?"

"Oh, Father, if you knew who I am you would never, never come to me," groaned Old Tom. "I am a vile sinner. I've committed an awful crime. God has forsaken me and He's right. What can I hope for but punishment, punishment, punishment!" he shouted more vehemently. He was evidently in an agony of fear and despair.

"Hush, Tom, said the priest consolingly. "What are you saying! God is good! He is long-suffering and merciful and forgiving. If you have done wrong, make your confession. God will forgive you, Tom. He is good."

"Oh, there is no hope for me. He will never forgive me—never! The dying man almost shrieked in his fear.

"Why should he not?" continued the priest. "Surely you are sorry. Are you not sorry, Tom?"

"Sorry?" moaned the beggar. "I've been sorry these thirty long years, ever since I did that awful crime. If you could listen, I must tell someone. My sin is always before me."

Then, in a broken voice, he poured into the kind priest's ears the story of his crime:

"It was during the Revolution: Thirty long years ago, I was the honored and respected butler of a rich and noble family. Then there came bloodshed. The rich were sought and executed. My master and mistress—oh, how kind they were to me—were hidden secretly away with their two daughters and their young son. I knew where. And he who would betray them would obtain their property and their wealth. Greed ate away at me. I betrayed them. I saw them carted away to execution by the revolutionists. I saw the bloody work as the heads of the master and mistress and of their two daughters were sliced away from their shoulders. The son alone was spared. A little boy . . . Pierre was his name." Here the priest stared intently at the old man. In his own heart he uttered a cry of agony and pain for that poor family. But the beggar, all absorbed in his recital, continued feverishly: "And oh, I keep seeing their faces before me. My God! My God! I keep seeing their blood—they were so kind to me, so kind. THERE THEY ARE BEHIND THAT CUR-

TAIN. There they have been hanging in that portrait for years—haunting me! haunting me!" And with this frantic, fearful cry, the miserable man fell back upon his pillow.

Father Pierre, somewhat shocked by the entire incident, pale and trembling, walked to the adjacent wall. He drew aside the ragged, soiled curtain that Tom had indicated. He stared intently upon the portrait of that noble family. There, in that portrait, stood a father and a mother, two daughters, and one little boy.

Allowing the curtain to drop to its normal hanging position, the priest returned to the bedside. He seated himself next to Old Tom. Calmly and softly he spoke: "Tom, God is good. Tom, confess now and all will be forgiven."

The power of grace filled that entire room. The spirit of God's love touched that wounded wretch. The old beggar copiously wept tears of repentance. From his weakened lips, dry and parched from his sickness, he muttered as clearly as possible his fervent confession.

"*Ego te absolvo a peccatis tuis:* I absolve you from your sins." In God's own name the words of absolution fell from the lips of the holy priest. The beggar was forgiven, reconciled and loved by his God.

"Now," said the priest, turning to the sinking man, "As God has forgiven you, so I also forgive you—WITH ALL MY HEART. Your master, Tom, was my father. Your mistress was my mother. Their daughters were my beloved sisters. I AM PIERRE—the son who was spared."

The dying man opened his eyes in shock. He stared into the eyes of Father Pierre, who was holding him in his arms. The old man was bewildered, confused. . . . Could this be? Hatred washed by love . . . sin cleansed by forgiveness . . . an embrace in place of rebuttal. . . . It was really true! Love was to conquer, love was to renew, love was to regenerate, love was to open heaven.

Love had healed!

Then the old man fell listlessly into the arms of Father Pierre. Old Tom, doubly forgiven, was dead to this earth but healed of his wounds by Him Who is the world's Divine Physician!